Antidepressants Pocket Guide

by

Shlomo Brook, M.D.

Edited and revised by: **Karolina Brook,**

Published by CreateSpace, First edition 2013

Acknowledgment

To my wife Justyna.

Contents

Preface

Depression is a common and debilitating condition, which affects approximately one in eight people in the US (1). In addition it is expected to be the second-leading cause of disability in the world by the year 2020 (2). Nearly 10% of all primary care office visits are related to depression (3). Untreated depression carries an increased risk of morbidity and mortality from general medical conditions (5). Medical care costs may significantly decreased in remitted patients. Patients recovered from depression have 49% lower medical costs in the year following their treatment compared with patients whose depression persisted (6).

Depression can be treated successfully and remission is the aim of depression treatment, as it is associated with a return of normal psychosocial function, lower rates of relapse, lower risk of suicide and alcohol or drug abuse, lack of disabling symptoms and overall a better prognosis (4). Unfortunately, up to 30% of the patients with major depression remain depressed after one year of treatment. I hope that this book will serve you as a useful guide for the treatment of your depressive patients.

Reference

1 RC Kessler, P Berglund, O Demler et al.: The epidemiology of MD: results from the national comorbiditysurvey replication (NCS-R). Jama 2003;289:3095-3105.

2 CJ Murray, AD Lopez. Global mortality, disability and the contribution of risk factors: Global burden of disease study. Lancet 1997;349:1436-1442.

3 RS Stafford, JC Ausiello, B Misra et al. national patterns of depression treatment in primary care. J Clin Psychiatry 2000; 2:211-216.

4 MH Trivedi, AJ Rush, SR Wisnieski et al. Evaluation of outcome with citalopram for depression. Am J Psychiatry 2006;163:28-40.

5 JM Zajecka. Treating depression to remission. J Clin Psychiatry 2003:64 (15):7-12.

6 GE Simon, D Reviki, J Heilitigenstein et al. Recovery from depression, work productivity, and health care costs among primary care patients. Gen Hosp Psychiatry 2000;22:153-162.

One
The clinical use of antidepressants

Over the past 50 years, antidepressants have become the principal treatment modality for moderate to severe depression. Furthermore, currently there is sufficient evidence to suggest that long-term use of antidepressants can significantly reduce the risk of recurrence, as well as improve the patient's quality of life and their level of functioning.

All currently available antidepressants have an average of 60% response rate after the treatment of depression. In addition, all antidepressants require at least one to three weeks of continuous use to demonstrate a response.

The British National Clinical Practice Guidelines (NICE guidelines) published in 2004 suggest that SSRIs should be the first-line of treatment for depression because they are as effective as TCAs, and their use is less likely to be discontinued due to their favorable side-effect profile (1).

However, data from 93 trials of dual-action antidepressants, suggests that the newer–generation antidepressants have a possible better response rate of 63% compared to the older SSRIs class which have a response rate of 59% (2,3).

A study conducted in 2009 by Cipriani et al, found that the response rates to mirtazapine, escitalopram, venlafaxine and sertraline were superior to that of duloxetine, fluoxetine, fluvoxamine and paroxetine(4).

However, sertraline, escitalopram and bupropion were, to a greater degree, better tolerated and more accepted by the patients than the rest of the antidepressants (4).

Residual symptoms of depression can predict recurrence (5). Follow-up studies with recovered patients found that 85% had a recurrence within 15 years (6). However, most studies showed that long-term use of antidepressants appear to prevent relapse (7).

Treatment strategies

Figure 1.1 shows a systematic strategy for the treatment of MDD

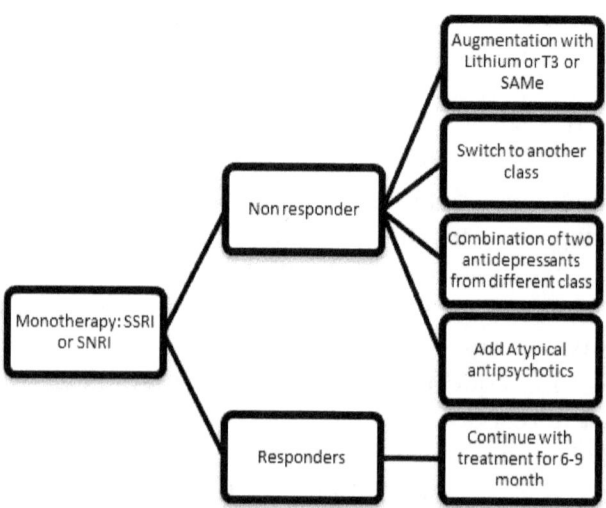

Figure 1.1: Antidepressant treatment strategies

Augmentation strategies

Lithium

In a multicenter double–blind randomized parallel group clinical trial on the efficacy of the combination of clomipramine 150mg/day plus lithium carbonate 750mg/day versus clomipramine 150mg/day plus placebo for the treatment of unipolar MDD, the patients with lithium augmentation showed a significant improvement of the depressive symptoms within the first week of treatment (8). In this study, 79% of the patients who received lithium augmentation responded to the combined lithium and clomipramine treatment while 71% of the patients on clomipramine and placebo responded. Such optimistic results were not replicated in the STAR*D study which was conducted in the US and published in 2008. The STAR*D study enrolled 4,041 nonpsychotic depressed outpatients at 23 psychiatric and 18 primary care sites. 2786 patients were randomized and received citalopram for 12-weeks.

After 12-weeks of treatment, non-responders were given either a different antidepressant or continued with citalopram augmented with bupropion or buspirone. Those patients who failed to respond were either switched to mirtazapine or placed subsequently, on Lithium carbonate augmentation or T3 augmentation (17).

The results of the STAR*D study showed that the augmentation with Lithium produced modest increase in response rates (9).

STAR*D Study design is illustrated in Figure 1.2

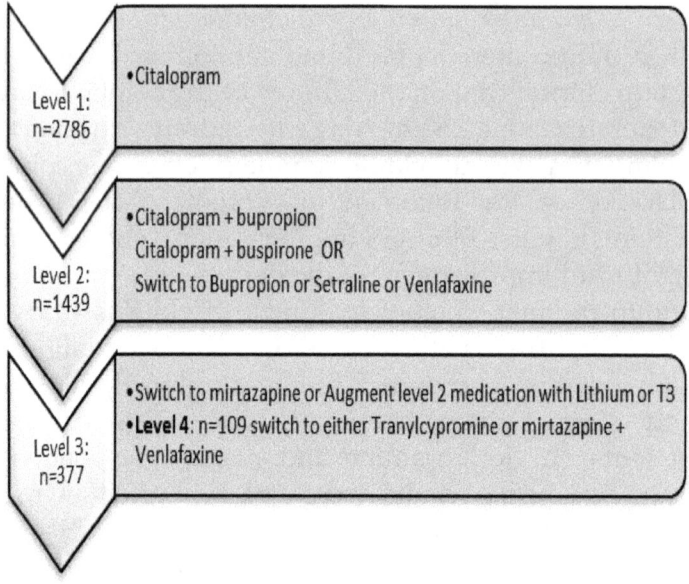

Figure 1.2 STAR*D study design

Thyroid Hormone (T3) augmentation

Early studies with Triiodothyronine (T3) showed some promise when it could improve depressive symptoms when augmented with antidepressants. However, in the STAR*D study the augmentation with T3 produced only a modest additional response rate (9). It appears that T3 is not likely to accelerate the clinical response to SSRIs in Major Depression (10).

SAMe

S-Adenosyl methionine (SAMe) was discovered in Italy by G.L Cantoni in 1952. SAMe is made from ATP and methionine and it is involved in numerous intracellular metabolic reactions as well as in cellular growth and repair.

SAMe is also involved in the biosynthesis of hormones and neurotransmitters, such as dopamine and serotonin.

SAMe is sold as a dietary supplement in a form of enteric-coated tablets. SAMe peak plasma concentration is reached in 3-5 hours and it has a half-life of 2 hours.

Early studies with S-adenosyl methionine (SAMe) showed some antidepressant promise, which led to consideration of its use as an augmentation to antidepressant medications. However, further studies are needed to explore the role of SAMe as an augmentation to antidepressant treatment.

Folic acid

Folic acid is the water soluble form of vitamin B9 and is essential for numerous bodily functions, such as DNA synthesis and repair, cell division and growth.

Leafy vegetables are the principal source of folic acid as humans are not able to synthesize folic acid.

Dietary low intake of Vitamin B9 may lead to folic acid deficiency which in developing embryos may result in neural tube defects while in adult it may cause macrocytic anemia peripheral neuropathy depression and cognitive impairment.

A recent study with 500mcg of folic acid augmentation to fluoxetine reported a 93% response rate, compared to only a 61% response rate in patients who were treated with fluoxetine alone (11).

Lamotrigine

Several small studies with lamotrigine augmentation showed some modest improvement in depressed patient's response rates when compared to placebo augmentation of antidepressants.

In a small double-blind randomized placebo-controlled trial of augmentation with lamotrigine 100mg or placebo in patients concomitantly treated with fluoxetine for resistant MDD, the lamotrigine augmented group showed statistical superiority to placebo on the Clinical Global Impression (CGI) Scale scores (12).

However, the benefit of using anticonvulsants as augmentation to antidepressants as first-line treatment for MDD is still questionable (13).

Atypical antipsychotics

A meta- analysis of randomized controlled trials with atypical antipsychotic augmentation in patients with MDD found that such augmentation was significantly more effective than placebo. Further, there were no differences in efficacy between olanzapine, risperidone, quetiapine or aripiprazole augmentation (14). However, the augmentation with atypical antipsychotics was associated with higher discontinuation rates due to side effects.

These included weight gain and metabolic syndrome, over sedation, fatigue, somnolence, hyperprolactinemia, and dyslipidemia as well as extrapyramidal side effects, including akathisia, dystonic reactions, Parkinsonism and tardive dyskinesia (13). In addition to safety and tolerability issues related to the atypical antipsychotic augmentation, the significant increase of cost merits additional consideration (2).

Antidepressant combination

It appears that the combination of two antidepressants with a different mode of action may increase the patient's response rates.
In a small double blind randomized study of antidepressant combination for the treatment of MDD (15), the combination of mirtazepine with fluoxetine, venlafaxine or bupropion was shown to produce statistically better remission rates than that of fluoxetine monotherapy.

The results of this study are shown in figure 1.3

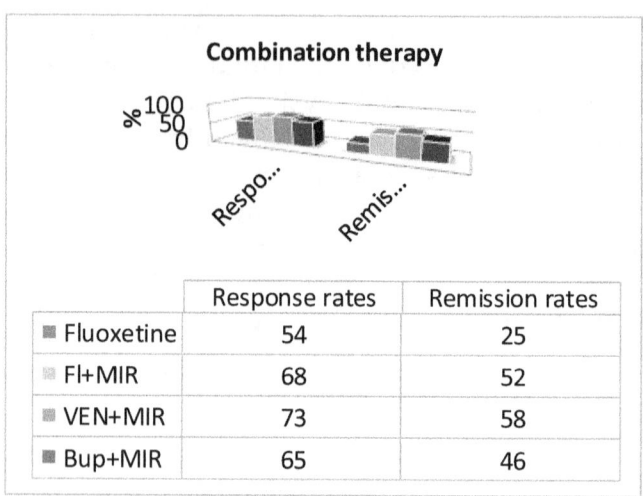

	Response rates	Remission rates
▪ Fluoxetine	54	25
▪ Fl+MIR	68	52
▪ VEN+MIR	73	58
▪ Bup+MIR	65	46

Figure 1.3 The various combination of mirtazapine (MIR), venlafaxine (VEN) or Bupropion (BUP) compared to fluoxetine (FL) monotherapy. Adapted from Blier P, Ward HE, Tremblay P et al. Combination of antidepressant medications from treatment initiation for MDD: a double blind randomized study. American Journal of Psychiatry. 2010, 167(3), 281-288.

The combination of antidepressants with different mode of action, particularly for the treatment resistant depressive patient may improve their response and remission rates. However, In addition to safety and tolerability issues related to the combination of two antidepressant medications, the significant increase in cost is an important consideration.

Modafinil

Modafinil is an agent approved by the FDA for the treatment of narcolepsy and shift work sleep disorder and as adjunctive treatment for obstructive sleep apnea syndrome. In a small randomized double-blind study (16), modafinil was added to SSRIs from the onset of treatment of MDD patients who also had fatigue and sleepiness. However, the combination of modafinil with SSRI did not show any significant improvement in the depressive symptoms over the group of patients treated only with SSRI.

The clinical use of antidepressants references

1 Nice guidelines 2004. Depression: Management of depression in primary and secondary care. National Clinical Practice Guidelines. Number 23. London: National Institute for clinical Excellence.

2 Stein D, Lerer B, Stahl SM: Essential Evidence – Based Psychopharmacology. Second edition. Cambridge University Press 2012.

3 Papakostas GI, Thase ME, Fava M et al: Are antidepressant drugs that combine serotonergic and noradrenergic mechanisms of action more effective than the SSRIs in treating MDD? A meta-analysis of studies of newer agents. Biological Psychiatry 2007;62:1217-1227.

4 Cipriani A, Furukawa TA, Salanti G et al. Comparative efficacy and acceptability of 12 new generation antidepressants: A multiple –treatment meta-analysis. Lancet 2009;373, 746-758.

5 Judd L, Akiskal HS, Maser JD et al. A prospective 12-years study of subsyndromal and syndromal depressive symptoms in unipolar MDD. J of Affective Disorder. 1998;50,97-108.

6 Mueller T, Leon AC, Keller MB et al. Recurrence after recovery from MDD during 15 years of observational follow up. American Journal of Psychiatry 1999,156;1000-1006.

7 Weiths KL, Houser T, Bately SR et al. Continuation phase treatment with bupropion SR effectively decreases the risk for relapse of depression. Biological Psychiatry. 2002, 51; 753-761.

8 Januel D, Poirier MF, D'alche-Biree F et al. Multicenter double – blind randomized parallel group clinical trial of efficacy of the combination clomipramine 150mg/day plus lithium 750mg/day versus clomipramine plus placebo in the treatment of unipolar MDD. Journal of Affective Disorder 2003;76(1-3), 191-200.

9 Rush AJ, Trivedi MH, Wisniewski SR et al. Acute and longer term outcomes in depressed outpatients requiring one or several treatment steps: A STAR*D report. American Journal of Psychiatry 2006, 163, 1905- 1917.

10 Papakostas GL, Cooper-Kazaz R, Appelhof BC et al. Simultaneous initiation of pharmacotherapy with T3 and SSRI for MDD. A quantitative synthesis of double-blind studies. International Clinical Psychopharmacology. 2009, 24(1), 19-25.

11 Coopen A Bailey J. Enhancement of the antidepressant action of fluoxetine by folic acid: A randomized, placebo controlled trial. Journal of Affective Disorders. 2000, 60(2), 121-130.

12 Barbosa L, Berk M, Voster M. A double-blind randomized placebo-controlled trial of augmentation with lamotrigine or placebo in patients concomitantly treated with fluoxetine for resistant MDD. Journal of Clinical Psychiatry 2003. 64, 403-407.

13. Papakostas GI, Fava M. Pharmacotherapy for depression and treatment resistant depression. World Scientific 2010.

14 Nelson JC, Papakostas GI. Atypical antipsychotic augmentation in MDD: A meta analysis of placebo-controlled randomized trials. American Journal of Psychiatry. 2009, 166, 980-991.

15 Blier P, Ward HE, Tremblay P et al. Combination of antidepressant medications from treatment initiation for MDD: a double blind randomized study. American Journal of Psychiatry. 2010, 167(3), 281-288.

16 Dunlop BW, Crits-Christoph P, Evans DL, et al. Co administration of modafinil and a SSRI from the initiation of treatment of MDD with fatigue and sleepiness: A double-blind, placebo controlled study. Journal of Clinical Psychopharmacology, 2007, 27(6), 614-619.

17 Warden D, Rush AJ, Trivedi Mh et al. The STAR*D Project results: A comprehensive review of findings. Curr. Psychiatry Rep. 2007, 9(6), 449-459.

Two
Agomelatine

Brand name: Valdoxane

Mode of action

- **Melatonin MT1 & MT2 receptors:** Agomelatine is a potent MT1 & MT2 Agonist.
- **Serotonin 5-HT2C receptors:** 5-HT2c antagonist.
- **Anticholinergic (Ach):**   No effects
- **Histaminergic (H1):**   No effects
- **Adrenergic α1:**   No effects

The melatonin MT1 and MT2 receptors

The majority of the MT1 receptors are located in the pituitary gland, and in the suprachiasmatic area of the hypothalamus. Activation of the MT1 receptors facilitates sleep, while the activation of the MT2 receptors, which are predominantly located in the retina, facilitate the phase shift circadian rhythms.

The activation of both MT1 and MT2 receptors result in re synchronization of the circadian rhythms, while the inhibition of the melatonin MT1 and MT2 receptors result in de-synchronization of the body's circadian rhythms.

Circadian rhythms are physical and mental changes that have a 24-hour cycle and are controlled by a master clock that consists of a group of nerve cells which are situated in the suprachiasmatic nucleus (SCN) located in the hypothalamus.

The presence or absence of light is the principal cue which influences and regulates the circadian rhythms.

The human circadian rhythms consist of the sleep – wake cycle, cortisol secretion, glucose homeostasis, metabolism and body temperature.

The circadian rhythms are controlled by two genes located in the suprachiasmatic nucleus (SCN): **BMAL1** and **Clock**. When both genes become active, they activate the expression of two intracellular proteins: **Per** and **Cry** which dimerize and then exit the nucleus and move into the cytoplasm. In the cell cytoplasm, the dimerized Per and Cry become phosphorylated and inhibit the BMAL1 and clock genes' expression via a negative feedback loop.

Once the phosphorylated Per and Cry proteins are degraded by a kinase the transcription of BMAL1 and Clock will start all over again. Light stimuli transmitted to the SCN via the retinohypotalamic tract affects the expression of the circadian rhythm central pacemaker. The SCN has high concentration of melatonin MT1 and MT2 as well as 5-HT2C receptors. The binding of melatonin to the MT1 and MT2 receptors in the SCN, suppresses neuronal firing and facilitates sleep. Melatonin supplement is used to facilitate the readjustment of the light – dark shifts that occurr in jet lag and shift work (2).

Abnormal circadian rhythm is associated with sleep disorders, depression and seasonal affective disorder.

Pharmacokinetics of agomelatine

Pharmacokinetics: **Linear pharmacokinetics**. Food intake does not modify the absorption rates and the bioavailability of agomelatine. Any dose change of agomelatine leads to a proportional change in agomelatine plasma levels

Tmax: 1-2 hours
Side effects may develop within 1 hours of agomelatine ingestion. Female and elderly patients may show higher plasma levels.

Absorption: >80%
Food may minimally slow agomelatine absorption.

Steady state: **5-7 days.**

Protein binding: **95%.** 35% is bound to albumin and 35% to acid glycoprotein.

Bioavailability: **<5%**

Half-life (t ½): **2-3 hours**

Metabolism: CYP 450 enzymes: **1A2**
                                                2C9
                                                2C19

Agomelatine has inactive metabolites: *hydroxylate agomelatine and 7-o-demethylated agomelatine.*

Elimination: **80% Urine**
                          20% Faeces

How supplied

- Tab of 25mg

Dose range

For major depressive disorder: 25-50mg as once daily dose given at bedtime.

How to stop treatment

A sudden discontinuation of agomelatine was not associated with discontinuation syndrome. However, a slow tapering of the drug is still recommended.

Clinical indications

- Major Depressive Disorder
- Generalized Anxiety Disorder
- Sleep disturbances

Side effects

CNS
- somnolence
- sedation
- fatigue
- headache
- Insomnia
- agitation
- anxiety
- **vivid dreams**
- dizziness
- **seizures** (very rare)
- rash

Gastrointestinal
- decreased appetite
- nausea ,
- vomiting
- dry mouth
- diarrhea
- constipation
- upper abdominal pain

Sexual
- decreased sex drive
- delayed ejaculation
- Impotence

- abnormal orgasm

Agomelatine serious side effects include

- Confusion
- Excitation
- Onset of seizure
- Yellow skin / eyes

- Fatigue
- Severe allergic reaction
- Irregular heart beats
- Hypertension
- Hypotension
- Induction of manic or hypomanic episode
- Activation of suicidal ideation and behaviour

Use during pregnancy

Safety unknown.

Equally important, the use of agomelatine in the last trimester of pregnancy may be associated with a higher incidence of respiratory distress and pulmonary hypertension, cyanosis, apnea, seizures, temperature instability, vomiting, hypoglycemia, hypotonia, hyperreflexia, tremor, irritability, constant crying and jitteriness, which may require prolonged hospitalization, tube feeding and respiratory support

Use during lactation

Secretion in the human breast milk is unknown

Agomelatine drug interactions

- **Drug interactions with Fluvoxamine: Increases** agomelatine plasma levels by 44 – fold.
- **Drug interaction with Omeprazole: Decreases** agomelatine blood levels.
- **Drug interaction with Paroxetine: Increases** agomelatine blood levels.
- **Drug interaction with Oestrogen: Increases** agomelatine blood levels.
- **Drug interaction with Tramadol**: Increases the risk to develop seizures.

Avoid using agomelatine in the following cases

- Concomitant use of MAOIs.
- Proven allergy to agomelatine.
- History of seizure.

Warnings for agomelatine

- **Pregnancy: Risk category unknown.**

- **Agomelatine may cause an increase in suicidal risk in young adults.** The use of antidepressants may increase the risk of suicidal thinking and behavior in children, adolescents and young adults aged 18-24.

- **Serotonin syndrome:** Symptoms may include agitation, dizziness, hallucinations, delirium, seizures and coma along with autonomic instability that includes tachycardia, fluctuating blood pressure, flushing, hyperthermia, tremor, muscular rigidity, myoclonus, hyperreflexia, incoordination.
- **Activation of hypomania or mania:** May occurred in agomelatine-treated bipolar patients.
- **Seizure:** The risk of seizure is relatively low with agomelatine.
- **Hepato–biliary disorder:** Agomelatine may increase the liver enzymes ALAT > 3 times the upper limit of the normal range. Liver function test should be performed in all patient at the initiation of treatment with agomelatine and then periodically after 3 weeks, 6 weeks, 12 weeks, and in 24 weeks. Any dose increase of agomelatine requires new liver function test to be performed at the same frequency as when initiating treatment. Any increase in serum transaminase requires urgent liver function test which must be repeated within 48hours.
- **Kidney impairment:** Agomelatine should be used with caution in patients with renal impairment and require a lower dose.
- **MAOI:** Agomelatine combined with MAOI may be fatal. Agomelatine requires 7 day washout period before starting with MAOI. Agomelatine requires 3 week washout period after MAOI was stopped.

- **Alcohol abuse:** Agomelatine is not recommended in patient abusing alcohol.

Agomelatine overdose

Overdose symptoms

- over sedation
- somnolence
- agitation
- anxiety
- tension
- dizziness
- fatigue
- disorientation
- seizure
- vomiting
- cyanosis
- loss of consciousness

How to manage agomelatine overdose

Agomelatine is relatively safe in mono therapy overdose.

In general, there is no antidote for agomelatine overdose and the management is mainly supportive, aimed to maintaining respiration, pulse and blood pressure. In the event of a recent overdose with agomelatine, a stomach washout, possibly with activated charcoal, may help to eliminate the un-absorbed drug and is done with large–bore oro-gastric tube, maintaining appropriate airway protection. In most cases, agomelatine overdose, requires to hospitalize the patient for at least 24 hours for intense observation

Agomelatine references

1 Stahl SM. Valdoxan: A novel antidepressant. Arbor Scientia 2011.

2 Arendt J, Skene DJ, Middleton B eta al. Efficacy of melatonin treatment in jet lag, shift work and blindness. J Biol Rhythms. 1997:12:604-617.

3 Stahl SM. Essential Psychopharmacology of depression and bipolar disorders. Cambridge University Press. 2000.

4 Kennedy SH, Emsley R. Placebo controlled trial of agomelatinein the treatment of MDD. Eur. Neuropsychopharmacology. 2006:16:93-100.

Three
Bupropion

Brand name: Wellbutrin

Mode of action

- **Norepinephrine Reuptake Transporters (NET): antagonist.**
- **Dopaminergic Reuptake Transporters (DAT): antagonist.**
- **Nicotinic receptors (α3β4):** Bupropion is a nicotinic acetylcholine receptors α3β4 **antagonist.**
- **Anticholinergic (Ach):**   Low affinity
- **Histaminergic (H1):**   Low affinity
- **Adrenergic (α1):**   Low affinity

Pharmacokinetics of bupropion

Pharmacokinetics: **Linear pharmacokinetics**. The higher the daily dose of bupropion, the higher the plasma level will get.

Peak plasma level (Tmax):
- IR Immediate release: **2-hours**
- XL formulation: **5 hours**.
- Bupropion metabolite: up to **43 hours**

Absorption: Bupropion is well absorbed by the gastrointestinal system and *it is not affected by the presence of food.*

Steady state: **8 days**.

Protein binding: **80%** mostly to albumin.

Bioavailability: Unknown. (**20%** in animals).

Half-life (t ½): **12-14 hours**

Metabolism: CYP 450 enzymes: **2B6**

2D6

Bupropion metabolizes into three major metabolites: *S-SHydroxybupropion, Threohyrobupropion and Erythrohydrobupropion.*

Out of the three metabolites, only the S-S hydroxybupropion has been shown to possess significant biological activity.

Bupropion's metabolism displays high variability. It appears that the metabolism of bupropion can vary up to 7-fold, in the same person, which can increase bupropion's half- life from 12 to 38 hours

Elimination: **80% Urine**
                  20% Faeces

How supplied

- Bupropion IR Tablets: 75mg, 100mg.
- Bupropion XL: 150mg, 300mg
- Bupropion SR: 100mg, 150mg, 200mg

Dose range

For major depressive disorder:
- **Bupropion XL**: 150mg – 450mg once daily.
- **Bupropion SR**: 200mg – 450mg in 2 divided doses.
- **Bupropion IR**: 150-450mg/day

How to treat

- **XL formula**: Start with bupropion XL 150mg once a day in the morning to be increase to 300mg once a day after 4 days. In severe cases, a maximum of 450mg can be given once daily.

How to stop treatment

Although there are no reports of withdrawal symptoms following bupropion cessation, a slow tapering of bupropion is recommended.

Clinical indications

- Major depression
- Nicotine addiction
- ADHD?

Side effects

Nervous system
- Agitation
- Insomnia
- Restlessness
- Muscle pain
- Tremor
- Hot flushes
- Headache
- Dizziness
- *Seizures* (more common in predisposed individuals and with immediate release formulation)
- Increased sweating
- Fatigue
- Somnolence
- Rash
- Blurred vision

Gastro intestinal System: Bupropion's GI side effects are highly common and can develop within 30 minutes of bupropion ingestion. They are more likely the result of the direct effect of bupropion on the intestinal mucosa than of its peak plasma level.

- *Decreased appetite*
- Weight loss
- Nausea
- Vomiting
- Dry mouth
- Diarrhea
- Constipation
- *Possible weight loss*
- Gastritis

Sexual: Bupropion use is associated with lower incidence of sexual dysfunction. Bupropion's most common sexual side effects are:

- Decreased sex drive
- Delayed ejaculation
- Impotence
- Abnormal orgasm

Bupropion's side effects that need immediate attention

- Confusion
- Excitation
- Onset of seizure
- Yellow skin / eyes
- Severe allergic reaction

- Irregular heart beats
- Hypertension
- Induction of manic or hypomanic episode
- Activation of suicidal ideation and behaviour

Bupropion discontinuation reaction

A sudden discontinuation of bupropion may be associated with a discontinuation reaction which is self-limiting. The most common symptoms of bupropion discontinuation reaction are:

- Irritability
- Agitation
- Dizziness
- Electric shock sensations
- Anxiety
- Confusion
- Headache
- Lethargy
- Insomnia
- Seizures
- Dysphoric mood

A slow down-titration of bupropion is often reduce the risk of having the discontinuation reaction.

Use during pregnancy: FDA risk category C (i.e.: some animal studies showed adverse effects but there are no controlled studies in humans). The use of bupropion in the last trimester of pregnancy may be associated with a higher incidence of respiratory distress and pulmonary hypertension, cyanosis, apnea, seizures, temperature instability, vomiting, hypoglycemia, hypotonia, hyperreflexia, tremor, irritability, constant crying and jitteriness, which may require prolonged hospitalization, tube feeding and respiratory support.

Use during lactation: Bupropion is secreted in the breast milk. Due to its unknown effects on the newborn's normal growth and development, breast feeding should be avoided.

Avoid using bupropion in the following cases

- Recent head injury
- History of seizure
- Current or past history of anorexia
- Current or past history of bulimia
- Alcohol withdrawal
- Brain tumor
- Proven allergy to bupropion
- MAOIs

Bupropion drug interactions

- **Drug interactions with L-Dopa: Increased** excitement, restlessness, nausea and tremor.

- **Drug interaction with Imipramine & Nortrityline: Increased** imipramine blood levels by 57%, and increased nortriptyline blood levels by 200%.
- **Drug interaction with Fluoxetine:** Delirium, panic and myoclonus.
- **Drug interaction with Venlafaxine:** 3-fold increase in the venlafaxine levels .
- **Drug interactions with MAOIs:** CNS toxicity-serotonin syndrome.
- **Drug interactions with Tramadol & Codeine:** Increased seizures risk and interfere with the analgesic action of codeine.
- **Drug interactions with Quinolone:** Seizures
- **Drug interactions with Zolpidem:** Hallucinations.
- **Drug interactions with Pseudoephedrine:** Seizures.
- **Drug interactions with Thioridazine:** Cardiac arrhythmias.
- **Drug interactions with Metropolol: Increases** metropolol blood levels.

Warnings for Bupropion

- **Pregnancy: Risk category C**
- **Alcohol abuse:** Bupropion is not recommended in patient abusing alcohol.

- **Bupropion may cause an increase in suicidal risk in young adults.** The use of antidepressants may increase the risk of suicidal thinking and behavior in children, adolescents and young adults aged 18-24.
- **Serotonin syndrome:** Symptoms may include agitation, dizziness, hallucinations, delirium, seizures and coma along with autonomic instability that includes tachycardia, fluctuating blood pressure, flushing, hyperthermia, tremor, muscular rigidity, myoclonus, hyperreflexia, incoordination.
- **Activation of hypomania or mania:** May occurred in bupropion-treated bipolar patients.
- **Seizure:** Bupropion immediate release carries a risk of seizure of 0.4% at doses below 450mg/day (which is 2-4 times higher than that of an SSRI). **Hypertension:** Bupropion has been reported to elevate blood pressure. **Kidney impairment:** Bupropion should be used with caution in patients with renal impairment and require a lower dose.
- **Liver impairment:** Bupropion should be avoided in patients with liver cirrhosis and liver insufficiency.
- **Heart disease:** Bupropion need to be used with caution in patients with cardiac impairment.

- **MAOI:** Bupropion with MAOI may be fatal. Bupropion requires 7 day washout period before starting with MAOI. Bupropion requires 3 week washout period after MAOI was stopped.
- **Elderly:** Bupropion needs a lower dose in the elderly.
- **Anorexia:** Bupropion should be avoided in patients with anorexia nervosa.

Bupropion overdose

Bupropion is **relatively safe in mono therapy overdoses** and has a rare incidence of fatalities. Seizure was reported to develop in up to 30% of overdose cases. Other prominent symptoms of overdose include hallucinations, loss of consciousness, sinus tachycardia, ECG changes, such as conduction disturbances, QRS prolongation, and arrhythmias.

Overdose symptoms

- **Seizure**
- **abnormal heart rhythm: tachycardia or bradycardia**
- **hallucinations**
- cardiac failure
- vomiting
- over sedation

- agitation
- loss of consciousness

How to manage bupropion overdosed patients

In general, there is no antidote for bupropion overdose and the management is mainly supportive, aimed to maintaining respiration, pulse and blood pressure. In the event of a recent overdose with bupropion, a stomach washout, possibly with activated charcoal, may help to eliminate the unabsorbed drug and is done with large–bore orogastric tube, maintaining appropriate airway protection. In most cases, bupropion overdose, requires to hospitalize the patient for at least 24 hours for intense observation.

Bupropion references

1. Eric J NestlerHyman S, Malenka, R. Moleculat neuropharmacology. A foundation for clinical neuroscience. Mcgraw Hill companies, Inc. 2001.

2. Zung WWK, Brodie HKH, Fabre L et al.: Comparative efficacy and safety of bupropion and placebo in the treatment of depression. Psychopharmacology (Berl) 1983,79:343-347.

Four
Citalopram

Brand name: Cipramil, Celexa

The s- isomer of citalopram have the brand names: **Lexapro, Cipralex** and have the following structural formula:

Mode of action

- **Serotonin Reuptake Transporters (SERT):** **antagonist.**
- **Anticholinergic (Ach):**   **Low affinity**
- **Histaminergic (H1):**   **Low affinity**
- **Adrenergic (α1):**   **Low affinity**

Pharmacokinetics of citalopram

Pharmacokinetics: **Linear pharmacokinetics**. A dose increase of citalopram and S-citalopram will lead to a proportionate increase in their plasma levels.

Peak plasma level (Tmax): 2-4 hours

Absorption: Citalopram is well absorbed by the gastrointestinal system, and its absorption is **not** affected by the presence of food.

Steady state: 7 days.

Protein binding: **80%** mostly to albumin.

Half-life (t ½):   **Citalopram 35 hours**.
                S- citalopram 27 – 32 hours

Metabolism: CYP 450 enzymes:
                Citalopram: 2C19, 3A4 , 2D6
                S-Citalopram: 2C19, 3A4

Citalopram principal metabolites are *demethylcitalopram* **(DCT)**, *didemethylcitalopram* **(DDCT)**, and *citalopram – N- oxide* as well as *deaminated propionic acid derivative.* **Citalopram metabolites are inactive** and have a plasma concentration of only 50% of that of the parent drug and a half-life of 50 hours.

Elimination: Mostly in the **Faeces**

How supplied

Citalopram
- Tablet: 10mg, 20mg, 40mg
- Capsules 10mg, 20mg, 40 mg

S-citalopram
- Tablet 5mg,10mg,20mg
- Capsules 5 mg, 10 mg, 20mg. oral solution 5mg/5ml.

Dose range

- 10mg – 50 mg for depression

Clinical indications

- Major Depression(MDD)
- Panic disorder (PD)
- Obsessive compulsive disorder (OCD)
- Premenstrual dysphoric syndrome (PMDD)
- Post Traumatic Stress Disorder (PTSD)
- Generalised anxiety disorder (GAD)

- Social anxiety disorder (SAD)

How to treat Major Depressive Disorder (MDD)

Citalopram & S-citalopram can be taken either in the morning or in the evening in a single daily dose

- **Citalopram:** Start with 20mg a day in a single morning dose. Wait at least two weeks to assess the clinical status before increasing the dose up to a maximum of 40mg a day. Citalopram can be administered in the morning or at night as a once-daily single dose.

- **S- citalopram**: Start with an initial dose of 10 mg of S-citalopram a day and increase up to 20 mg/day if needed. S-citalopram can be administered in the morning or at night as a daily single dose.

In general, 10 mg of s-citalopram is comparable to 40 mg of citalopram and appeared to have a fewer side effects.

How to stop treatment

Due to their short half-life, and the possibility to develop withdrawal syndrome, upon abrupt discontinuation, a slow tapering off citalopram & S-Citalopram is strongly recommended.

Side effects

Nervous system

- insomnia
- agitation
- restlessness, jitteriness anxiety
- tremor
- increased sweating/ flushing
- headache
- dizziness
- seizures (rare)
- somnolence
- sedation
- fatigue
- cognitive slowing
- reduced attention
- apathy
- emotional blunting
- rash

Gastro intestinal: The GI side effects are common with citalopram and usually develop within 30 minutes of citalopram ingestion.

The GI side effects are more likely the result of the direct effect of citalopram on the intestinal mucosa. The most common GI adverse effects are:

- decreased appetite upper gastrointestinal symptoms
- nausea,
- vomiting,
- dry mouth
- diarrhea
- constipation
- possible weight loss

Sexual: The incidence of the sexual side effects with SSRIs use develops in 20 % - 40% of treated patients. Citalopram sexual side effects are dose dependent and do not diminish over time. However, most of the citalopram sexual side effects disappear upon treatment discontinuation.

The most common citalopram sexual side effects are:

- decreased sex drive
- delayed ejaculation
- impotence
- inability to reach an orgasm

Suicide

The FDA requires all antidepressants to carry a black box warning stating that antidepressant may increase the risk for suicide in persons under the age of 25 years.

This warning is based on data suggesting that suicidal ideations and behaviour has a 2-fold increase in children and in adolescents, and 1.5–fold increase in the 18 – 24 age group.

Citalopram side effects that need immediate attention

- Confusion
- Excitation
- Onset of seizure
- Yellow skin / eyes
- Severe allergic reaction
- Irregular heart beats Arrhythmia
- Low blood pressure
- Bruising and bleeding (relatively rare)
- Induction of manic episode
- Activation of suicidal ideation and behaviour

Citalopram discontinuation symptoms are

- Electric shock sensation
- insomnia
- dizziness
- light-handedness
- vertigo
- irritability
- bladder control problems
- akathisia: inability to stand still -
- Anxiety

A slow down-titration of citalopram is often reduces the risk of having the discontinuation reaction.

Use during pregnancy: FDA risk category C (i.e.: some animal studies showed adverse effects but there are no controlled studies in humans). The use of citalopram in the last trimester of pregnancy may be associated with a higher incidence of respiratory distress and pulmonary hypertension, cyanosis, apnea, seizures, temperature instability, vomiting, hypoglycemia, hypotonia, hyperreflexia, tremor, irritability, constant crying and jitteriness, which may require prolonged hospitalization, tube feeding and respiratory support.

Use during lactation: Citalopram and S-citalopram are secreted in the breast milk. Due to theirs unknown effects on the newborn's normal growth and development, breast feeding should be avoided.

Avoid using citalopram in the following cases

- Proven allergy to citalopram
- Concomitant use with MAOIs
- **Recently the FDA issued a warning for citalopram use to be limited to a maximum of 40 mg a day due to its ability to cause abnormal changes in the heart electrical activities such as QTC prolongation that can lead to cardiac arrhythmias.**

Citalopram drug interactions

- **Drug interactions with Warfarin:** Increased risk for risk of bleeding. Protrombin time was increased by 5%.
- **Drug interaction with Metropolol:** Increased metoprolol blood levels by 100%.
- **Drug interaction with Tramadol: Seizures**.
- **Drug interaction with Sumatriptan:** eakness and hyperreflexia and incoordination.
- **Drug interactions with MAOIs:** CNS toxicity-serotonin syndrome.
- **Drug interactions with Ketoconazole:** Decreased ketoconazole Cmax by 21%.
- **Drug interactions with Carbamazepine:** increase the clearance of citalopram

Warnings for citalopram

- **Pregnancy: Risk category C**

- **Citalopram may cause an increase in suicidal risk in young adults.** The use of antidepressants may increase the risk of suicidal thinking and behavior in children, adolescents and young adults aged 18-24.
- **Elderly**: Citalopram need a lower dose when it is used in patients above 60 years.

- **Serotonin syndrome:** Symptoms may include agitation, dizziness, hallucinations, delirium, seizures and coma along with autonomic instability that includes tachycardia, fluctuating blood pressure, flushing, hyperthermia, tremor, muscular rigidity, myoclonus, hyperreflexia, incoordination.
- **Activation of hypomania or mania:** May occurred in 0.2% of citalopram-treated bipolar patients.
- **Seizure:** Citalopram carries a risk of seizure of 0.3%.
- **Hyponatremia** may develop subsequent to the use of citalopram, especially in volume-depleted patients and in patients on diuretics.
- **Angle – closure glaucoma**: Citalopram may have an effect on the pupil size resulting in mydriasis.
- **Abnormal bleeding** was observed in patients using citalopram.
- **Liver impairment**: Citalopram needs a lower dose when it is used in patients with moderate liver impairment.

- **MAOI:** Combination of citalopram with MAOI may be fatal. Citalopram requires 7 day washout period before starting with MAOI. Citalopram requires 3 week washout period after MAOI was stopped.
- **Alcohol abuse:** Citalopram is not recommended in patient abusing alcohol.

Citalopram overdose

Citalopram & S-Citalopram are **rarely lethal in monotherapy overdose**. However, the concomitant use of citalopram with alcohol and/or with other central nervous depressants such as painkillers or benzodiazepines may result in death cause by respiratory depression.

Overdose symptoms

The most common symptoms of citalopram over dose are:
- nausea
- vomiting
- over sedation
- somnolence
- agitation
- abnormal heart rhythm: sinus tachycardia
- QTc prolongation
- dizziness
- sweating
- tremor
- convulsions
- amnesia
- confusion
- seizures
- cyanosis
- rabdomyolysis
- coma

How to manage citalopram overdosed patients

In general, there is no antidote for citalopram overdose and the management is mainly supportive, aimed to maintaining respiration, pulse and blood pressure. In the event of a recent overdose with citalopram, a stomach washout, possibly with activated charcoal, may help to eliminate the un-absorbed drug and is done with large–bore oro-gastric tube, maintaining appropriate airway protection. In most cases citalopram overdose, requires to hospitalize the patient for at least 24 hours for intense observation.

Citalopram references

1 Trivedi M, Rush AJ, Wisniewski SR et al. Evaluation of outcome with citalopram for depression using measurement – based care in STAR*D: implications for clinical practice. Am J Psychiatry Januarry 2006;163:1.

Five

Clomipramine

Brand name: Anafranil

Mode of action

- **Serotonine Re Uptake Transporters (SERT):** Antagonist.
- **Norepinephrine Re Uptake Transporters (NET):** Desmethylclomipramine (DMI), which is clomipramine's active metabolite, is a **strong antagonist** of the (NET).
- **Anticholinergic (Ach):**   **High affinity**
- **Histaminergic (H1):**   **Moderate affinity**
- **Adrenergic (α1):**   **High affinity**

Pharmacokinetics of clomipramine

Pharmacokinetics: Linear pharmacokinetics. A dose increase of clomipramine will lead to a proportionate increase in their plasma levels.

Peak plasma level (Tmax): 2-6 hours

Absorption: Clomipramine is well absorbed by the gastrointestinal system, and its absorption is **not** affected by the presence of food.

Steady state: 7-14 days.

Protein binding: **98%** mostly to albumin and to α1glycoprotein.

Half-life ($t\frac{1}{2}$**): 32 hours** for the parent drug.
                        69 hours for the active metabolite (DMI).

Bioavailability 50%

Metabolism: CYP 450 enzymes: : **2D6 and 1A2**

Elimination: **Urine 60%**
                        Faeces 30%

How supplied

- Clomipramine capsules of 25mg, 50mg, 75mg
- Clomipramine CR 75 mg.

Dose range

- Clomipramine 100 mg – 200mg a day for depression
- Clomipramine CR 75mg – 150mg a day for depression

Clinical indications

- Major depression
- Treatment resistant depression
- Anxiety
- Neuropathic pain
- Premature ejaculation
- Enuresis (involuntary nightly urination during sleep) in children and adolescents.
- Cataplexy syndrome

How to treat Major Depressive Disorder (MDD)

- **For Major Depression (MDD): S**tart with clomipramine 25mg, preferably at bedtime, and slowly increase the dose by increments of 25mg every 3 days up to a maximum of 200mg taken at bedtime in order to avoid excessive daily sedation.

- **For OCD:** Start with clomipramine 25mg once a day at bedtime to be increased every 3 days by increments of 25 mg up to a maximum dose of 250mg.

How to stop treatment

It is highly recommended to slowly taper clomipramine in order to minimize the emergence of withdrawal symptoms, which usually develops within the first 2 weeks of treatment cessation.
Clomipramine requires a 50% dose reduction every third day.

Side effects

Nervous system
- drowsiness
- lethargy
- fatigue
- weakness
- dizziness
- insomnia
- nausea
- blurred vision
- headache and worsening of migraine
- In coordination
- tremor
- disturbed concentration
- disorientation
- confusion
- restlessness and agitation (rare)
- *seizures* (clomipramine has the highest incidence among all TCAs to cause seizures especially in predisposed individuals. The

incidence of seizure in patients on clomipramine is 2% at doses above 300mg a day.
- stuttering
- disturbance in gait
- worsening of parkinsonism
- rash (rare)

Cardiac
- hypotension
- syncope
- bradycardia

Gastro intestinal
The gastro intestinal side effects can develop within 30 minutes of drug ingestion, and they are more likely the result of clomipramine anticholinergic effects.
- *decreased appetite*
- *heartburn*
- **weight gain (in 18% of patients)**
- nausea
- vomiting
- dry mouth
- constipation
- gastritis

Sexual
- decreased libido
- Impotence
- retrograde ejaculation

- painful ejaculation
- delayed ejaculation

Practical implication: due to its strong anticholinergic effects, clomipramine can be used for the treatment of premature ejaculation.

Suicide

The FDA requires all antidepressants to carry a black box warning stating that antidepressants may increase the risk for suicide in persons under the age of 25 years. This warning is based on data suggesting that suicide ideations and behavior has a 2-fold increase in children and in adolescents, and 1.5 – fold increase in the 18 – 24 age group.

Clomipramine Side effect that requires immediate attention

- Confusion
- Excitation
- Onset of seizure
- Yellow skin /eye
- Severe allergic reaction
- Irregular heart beats
- Hypotension
- Induction of manic or hypomanic episode
- Activation of suicidal ideation and behaviour especially in children and adolescents

Discontinuation symptoms

A sudden discontinuation of clomipramine may be associated with a discontinuation reaction. The discontinuation symptoms are usually self-limiting. The most common symptoms of clomipramine discontinuation reaction are:

- irritability
- agitation
- dizziness
- anxiety
- confusion
- headache
- lethargy
- insomnia
- seizures
- dysphoric mood
- fever
- fatigue
- sweating
- myalgia (muscle pain)

A slow down titration of clomipramine is often associated with a reduced risk of having the discontinuation reaction

Use during pregnancy: FDA risk category C (i.e.: some animal studies showed adverse effects but there are no controlled studies in humans). The use of clomipramine in the last trimester of pregnancy may be associated with a higher incidence of respiratory distress and pulmonary hypertension, cyanosis, apnea, seizures, temperature instability, vomiting, hypoglycemia, hypotonia, hyperreflexia, tremor, irritability, constant crying and jitteriness, which may require prolonged hospitalization, tube feeding and respiratory support.

Use during lactation: Clomipramine is secreted in the breast milk. Due to its unknown effects on the newborn's normal growth and development, breast feeding should be avoided.

Avoid using clomipramine in the following cases

- **Myocardial infraction**: patients recovering from myocardial infraction should avoid using clomipramine due to its propensity to cause cardiac arrhythmias, prolongation of conduction time and hypotension.
- **Hyperthyroidism:** Patients with hyper active thyroid gland are more sensitive to the clomipramine side effects.
- **Cardiac arrhythmia**: Patients with pre-existing cardiac disease and cardiac arrhythmias should be closely monitored and preferably avoid the use of clomipramine.

- History of seizure
- Prostate hypertrophy
- Pre-existing closed angle glaucoma
- Proven allergy to clomipramine

Clomipramine drug interactions

- **Drug interactions with Warfarin: Increased** risk for risk of bleeding.
- **Drug interaction with Carbamazepine: Decreses** clomipramine's blood levels.
- **Drug interaction with Tramadol: Seizures**.
  - **Drug interaction with Phenobarbital:** Increase phenobarbital blood level
  - **Drug interactions with MAOIs:** CNS toxicity-serotonin syndrome.
  - **Drug interactions with Akineton:** Increase anticholinergic effects.
  - **Drug interactions with Ketoconazole:** increase clomipramine's blood levels.
  - **Drug interactions with Fluoxetine: Increase clomipramine blood levels.**
  - **Drug interactions with Methylphenidate: Increase** clomipramine blood levels.
  - **Drug interactions with Cimetidine: Increase** clomipramine blood concentration.
  - **Drug interactions with Fluvoxamine: Increase** clomipramine blood concentration.
  - **Drug interaction with Grape fruit juice: Decrease** clomipramine metabolism.

Warnings for clomipramine

- **Pregnancy: Risk category C**

- **Clomipramine may cause an increase in suicidal risk in young adults.** The use of antidepressants may increase the risk of suicidal thinking and behavior in children, adolescents and young adults aged 18-24.
- **Serotonin syndrome:** Symptoms may include agitation, dizziness, hallucinations, delirium, seizures and coma along with autonomic instability that includes tachycardia, fluctuating blood pressure, flushing, hyperthermia, tremor, muscular rigidity, myoclonus, hyperreflexia, incoordination.
- **Activation of hypomania or mania:** may occurred in clomipramine treated bipolar patients.
- **Seizure:** The incidence of seizure in patients on clomipramine at doses of 300mg was 1.5%.
- **Cardiac impairment** clomipramine need to be used with caution in patients with cardiac impairment.
- **Angle – closure glaucoma**: Clomipramine may have an effect on the pupil size resulting in mydriasis.
- **Status post MI**: Clomipramine should be avoided in a patient with a recent myocardial infarct.
- **Renal impairment**: Clomipramine requires a dose adjustment (lower dose) in patients with mild to moderate renal impairment.

- **Elderly**: Citalopram need a lower dose when it is used in patients above 60 years.

- **Liver impairment**: Clomipramine must be avoided in patients with liver insufficiency. Clomipramine was associated with SGOT and SGPT elevation 3 times greater than the normal upper limit in up to 3% of treated patients.

- **MAOI:** Combination of clomipramine with MAOI may be fatal. Clomipramine requires 7 day washout period before starting with MAOI. Clomipramine requires 3 week washout period after MAOI was stopped.

- **Alcohol abuse:** Clomipramine is not recommended in patient abusing alcohol.

- **Urinary retention**: Clomipramine may worsen urinary retention in predisposed patients due to its anticholinergic properties.

- **Hyperthyroidism:** Clomipramine cardiac toxicity may be increased in patients with hyperthyroidism or in patients on thyroid medications.

- **Adrenal medulla tumours:** Clomipramine use in patients with adrenal tumours such as pheochromocytoma or neuroblastoma may be associated with hypertensive crisis.

- **Hematologic changes**: Clomipramine may be associated with leukopenia, agranulocytosis, thrombocytopenia, anemia, and pancytopenia. Leukocyte and differential blood count should be obtained in patients treated with clomipramine who develop fever and sore throat.

- **Hyperthermia**: Clomipramine was associated with hyperthermia especially when it was used in combination with other serotoninergic drugs.

Clomipramine overdose

Clomipramine may be lethal in mono therapy overdose. As a general rule, the bigger the amount of clomipramine ingested, the worse the reaction will get and the higher the possibility for lethal results.. However, the concomitant use of clomipramine with alcohol and/or with other central nervous depressants such as painkillers or benzodiazepines may result in death cause by respiratory depression.

Overdose symptoms

The most common symptoms of clomipramine over dose are:

- over sedation
- drowsiness
- respiratory depression
- cyanosis
- respiratory arrest
- seizure
- abnormal heart rhythm – mainly tachycardia

- ECG changes – particularly in QRS axis
- congestive heart failure
- cardiac arrest
- hypotension
- hyperactive reflexes
- muscle rigidity
- coreiform movements
- mydriasis
- oliguria
- anuria
- vomiting
- delirium
- loss of consciousness

How to manage clomipramine overdosed patients

In general, there is no antidote for clomipramine overdose and the management is mainly supportive, aimed to maintaining respiration, pulse and blood pressure.

In the event of a recent overdose with clomipramine, a stomach washout, possibly with activated charcoal, may help to eliminate the un- absorbed drug and is done with large–bore oro-gastric tube, maintaining appropriate airway protection. In most cases clomipramine overdose, requires to hospitalize the patient for at least 24 hours for intense observation.

Clomipramine references

1 LepineJP, Goger J, Blashko C. A double blind study of the efficacy and safety of sertraline and clomipramine in outpatients with severe MDD> Int Clin Psychoparmacol 2000 Sep.; 15(5):263-271.

2 Albert V, Aguglia E, Maina G. Venlafaxine versus clomipramine in the treatment of OCD. A preliminary single-blind 12 weeks controlled study. J Clin Psychiatry, Nov 2002:63(11):1004-1011.

3 Danish university antidepressant group. Citalopram clinical effect profile in comparison with clomipramine. A controlled multicentre study. Psychopharmacology, 1986, 90, 131-138.

4 Danish university antidepressant group. Comparative efficacy of clomipramine versus paroxetine in endogenous MDD. Journal of Affective Disorders, 1990,18,289-299.

Six

Duloxetine

Brand name: Cymbalta, Cymgen

Mode of action

- Duloxetine is a Serotonin Reuptake Transporter (SERT) antagonist.
- Duloxetine is a Norepinephrine Reuptake Transporter (NET) antagonist.
- Duloxetine is a Dopamine Reuptake Transporter (DAT) Antagonist.
- Duloxetine is an antagonist of serotonin receptors: 5-HT1A, 5-HT1B, 5 – HT1D, 5-HT2A and 5-HT2C.

- **Anticholinergic (Ach): Low affinity**
- **Histaminergic (H1): Low affinity**
- **Adrenergic (α1): Low affinity**

Pharmacokinetics of duloxetine

Pharmacokinetics: Linear pharmacokinetics. A dose increase of duloxetine will lead to a proportionate increase in its plasma levels.

Peak plasma level (Tmax): 6 hours

Absorption: Duloxetine is well absorbed by the gastrointestinal system. There is a 2-3 hours lag until absorption begins (Tlag=3H). The presence of food in the stomach may prolong the time needed to reach peak plasma concentration to between 6 to 10 hours.

Steady state: 3 days.

Protein binding: **95%** mostly to albumin and to α1glycoprotein..

Half-life (t ½): 12 hours

Bioavailability: 50%

Metabolism: CYP 450 enzymes: **2D6 and 1A2**
The principal plasma metabolites of duloxetine are the *4- hydroxy duloxetine glucuronide* and the *5-hydroxy, 6 - methyl duloxetine sulphate,* both clinically inactive.

Elimination: **Urine 70%**
Faeces 20%

How supplied

- Capsule   20mg, 30mg, 60 mg.

Dose range

- 30 mg – 60 mg for depression
- 60mg a day for diabetic peripheral neuropathic pain
- 60 mg for fibromyalgia
- 60 mg once a day for generalized anxiety disorder
- 40mg twice a day for stress urinary incontinence

Clinical indications

- Major depression
- Generalised anxiety disorder
- Diabetic peripheral neuropathic pain
- Stress urinary incontinence
- Fibromyalgia
- Chronic muscular pain

How to treat with duloxetine

- **For Major Depression (MDD)**: Start with 30 mg a day to be increased up to a maximum of 120mg a day.

- **For generalized anxiety disorder (GAD)**: Start with 30mg to be increased weekly up to a maximum of 120mg a day.

- **For fibromyalgia and neuropathic pain**: Start with 30 mg a day to be increased to a maximum of 60 mg a day. Doses above 60mg were associated with increased side effects.

How to stop treatment

Due to its relative short half-life, there is a need for a slow tapering of duloxetine in order to avoid withdrawal symptoms.

Side effects

Nervous system
- Insomnia
- Restlessness
- Restless leg syndrome
- Muscle spasm
- Tremor
- Hot flushes
- Headache
- Dizziness
- Seizures (rare and is mainly associated with upon treatment discontinuation)
- Increased sweating

- Fatigue
- Somnolence
- Rash

Psychiatric
- Lethargy
- Dyskinesia
- Myoclonus
- Poor sleep
- Increases stage 3 sleep
- Suppresses rapid eye movement (REM) sleep
- Paraesthesia
- Disturbed attention

Cardiac
- Palpitation
- Myocardial infraction
- Tachycardia

Gastro intestinal

GI symptoms are highly prominent with duloxetine use. The gastro intestinal side effects can develop within 30 minutes of drug ingestion, and they are more likely the result of the direct effect of duloxetine on the intestinal mucosa rather then the plasma peak level.

- Decreased appetite
- Nausea
- Vomiting

- Dry mouth
- Diarrhea
- Constipation
- Possible weight loss
- Gastritis

Sexual manifestations
The effects of duloxetine on sexual functioning are probably related to its effects on serotonin and are more prominent in males than in females.

- Decreased sex drive
- Delayed ejaculation
- Impotence
- Abnormal orgasm

Renal
- Dysuria
- Nocturia
- Polyuria
- Micturition urgency
- Abnormal urine odor

Musculoskeletal
- Musculoskeletal pain
- Muscle twitching

Eye manifestation
- Diplopia
- Visual disturbance
- Blurred vision

Suicide

The FDA requires all antidepressants to carry a black box warning stating that antidepressants may increase the risk for suicide in persons under the age of 25 years. This warning is based on data suggesting that suicide ideations and behavior has a 2-fold increase in children and in adolescents, and 1.5 – fold increase in the 18 – 24 age group.

Duloxetine side effects that requires immediate attention

- Confusion
- Excitation
- Onset of seizure
- Yellow skin / eye
- Severe allergic reaction
- Irregular heart beats
- Hypertension
- Induction of manic or hypomanic episode
- Activation of suicidal ideation and behaviour

Discontinuation symptoms

A sudden discontinuation of duloxetine may be associated with a discontinuation reaction. The discontinuation symptoms are usually self-limiting. The most common symptoms of duloxetine discontinuation reaction are:

- Irritability
- Agitation

- Dizziness
- Electric shock sensations
- Anxiety
- Confusion
- Headache
- Lethargy
- Insomnia
- Seizures
- Dysphoric mood

A slow down titration of duloxetine is often reduces the risk of having the discontinuation reaction.

Use during pregnancy: FDA risk category C (i.e.: some animal studies showed adverse effects but there are no controlled studies in humans). The use of duloxetine in the last trimester of pregnancy may be associated with a higher incidence of respiratory distress and pulmonary hypertension, cyanosis, apnea, seizures, temperature instability, vomiting, hypoglycemia, hypotonia, hyperreflexia, tremor, irritability, constant crying and jitteriness, which may require prolonged hospitalization, tube feeding and respiratory support.

Use during lactation: Duloxetine secreted in the breast milk. Duloxetine is secreted in the breast milk of lactating woman. The estimated daily infant dose is approximately 0.14% of that of the maternal dose. Due to its unknown effects on the newborn's normal growth and development, breast feeding should be avoided.

Avoid using duloxetine in the following cases

- History of seizure
- Prostate hypertrophy
- Proven allergy to duloxetine

Duloxetine drug interactions

- **Drug interactions with Warfarin: Increased** risk for risk of bleeding.
- **Drug interaction with fluvoxamine:** 2.5-fold increase in duloxetine peak plasma concentration and 3 fold increase in duloxetine half- life.
- **Drug interaction with zolpidem:** Delirium.
- **Drug interactions with MAOIs:** CNS toxicity-serotonin syndrome.
- **Drug interactions with Beta Blocker:** Increase duloxetine's plasma levels.
- **Drug interactions with Paroxetine:** increase duloxetine's AUC by 60%.
- **Drug interactions with Fluoxetine: Increase** duloxeine blood levels.
- **Drug interactions with triptans:** Serotonin-syndrome.
- **Drug interactions with lithium:** Serotonin syndrome.

- **Drug interactions with tramadol:** Serotonin syndrome.
- **Drug interaction with St John's wort:** Serotonin syndrome.

Warnings for Duloxetine

- **Pregnancy: Risk category C**

- **Duloxetine may cause an increase in suicidal risk in young adults.** The use of antidepressants may increase the risk of suicidal thinking and behavior in children, adolescents and young adults aged 18-24.
- **Serotonin syndrome:** Symptoms may include agitation, dizziness, hallucinations, delirium, seizures and coma along with autonomic instability that includes tachycardia, fluctuating blood pressure, flushing, hyperthermia, tremor, muscular rigidity, myoclonus, hyperreflexia, incoordination.
- **Activation of hypomania or mania:** May occurred in 0.1% of duloxetine treated bipolar patients.
- **Seizure:** The incidence of seizure in patients on duloxetine at doses of 300mg was 0.03%.
- **Syncope:** orthostatic hypotension and syncope have been reported with duloxetine mostly in the first week of treatment or after duloxetine dose increases.
- **Bleeding**: Duloxetine may increase the risk of bleeding especially whenever it is used with

- aspirin, warfarin and non-steroidal anti–inflammatory (NSAIDs) drugs.
- **Urinary hesitancy**: Duloxetine's ability to potentiate norepinephrine (NE) may increase urethral resistance which may cause urinary hesitancy.
- **Mydriasis:** Duloxetine should be avoided in patients having uncontrolled narrow-angle glaucoma.
- **Diabetes**: Duloxetine may worsen glycemic control in diabetic patients.
- **Hypertension:** Duloxetine treatment was associated with mean increase of 0.5mmHg in systolic blood pressure and 0.8mm Hg in diastolic blood pressure.
- **Renal impairment**: Duloxetine **does not** require any dose adjustment in mild to moderate renal impairment.
- **Alcohol:** Duloxetine is not recommended in patients abusing alcohol.
- **Thioridazine:** Duloxetine must be avoided in patients who are using Thioridazine.
- **MAOI:** Combination of duloxetine with MAOI may be fatal. Duloxetine requires 7 day washout period before starting with MAOI. Duloxetine requires 3 week washout period after MAOI was stopped.

Duloxetine overdose

Duloxetine is **relatively safe in mono-therapy overdose.** As a general rule, the bigger the amount of duloxetine ingested, the worse the reaction will get and the higher the possibility for lethal results.. However, the concomitant use of duloxetine with alcohol and/or with other central nervous depressants such as painkillers or benzodiazepines may result in death cause by respiratory depression.

Overdose symptoms
The most common symptoms of duloxetine over dose are:
- vomiting
- somnolence, over sedation
- agitation
- dilated pupils
- abnormal heart rhythm
- hypotension/ hypertension
- syncope
- tachycardia
- seizures
- coma

How to manage duloxetine's overdosed patients: In general, there is no antidote for duloxetine overdose and the management is mainly supportive, aimed to maintaining respiration, pulse and blood pressure. In the event of a recent overdose with duloxetine, a stomach washout, possibly with activated charcoal, may help to eliminate the un- absorbed drug and is done with large–bore oro-gastric tube, maintaining appropriate airway protection. In most cases duloxetine overdose, requires to hospitalize the patient for at least 24 hours for intense observation.

Duloxetine references

1 Thase M.E, Pritchett, Y.L, Ossana, M.J et al. Efficacy of duloxetine and SRI: comparisons as assessed by remission rates in patients with MDD. Journal of clinical Psychopharmacology, 2007;27(6), 672-676.

2 Goldstein DJ, Lu, Y, Derke MJ et al. Duloxetine in the treatment of depression: a double blind placebo – controlled comparison with paroxetine. J. Clin Psychopharmacol 2004 24 389 – 399.

3 Stahl SM, Megan M., Grady BA et al. SNRIs Their pharmacology, clinical efficacy and tolerability in comparison with other classes of antidepressants. CNS spectrum 2005;volume 10 number 9 732 – 747.

4 Zao R.,Cao J.,Peng W. In vitro and in vivo evaluation of the effects of duloxetine on P-gp function. Human Psychopharmacology Clinical And Experimental. 2010;Volume 25,issue 7-8, 553-559.

5 Mariapan P, Ballantyne Z., N'Dow JM. Cochrane database Syst Rev. 2005;(3): CD 004742.

6 Shamliyan TA, Kane RL, Wyman J. et al. Systematic review: randomized controlled trials of nonsurgical treatments for urinary incontinence in woman. Ann. Intern. Med. 2008;148 (6): 459 – 473.

7 Trial 2615A efficacy and safety of duloxetine compared with placebo, pelvic floor muscle training in subjects with moderate to severe stress urinary incontinence.
www.clinicalstudyresults.org/drugdetails/viewfile. php?.

8 Allgulander, C, Hartford, J, Russell, J. et al. Pharmacotherapy of GAD. Results of duloxetine treatment from pooled of three clinical trials. Urrent Medical and research opinion, 2007;23(6), 1245 – 1252.

Seven

Fluoxetine

Brand name: Prozac

Mode of action

- Fluoxetine is a Serotonin Reuptake Transporter (SERT) antagonist.
- Fluoxetine is a 5-HT2c antagonist.
- Fluoxetine desensitizes the 5-HT1A auto-receptor.
- Anticholinergic (Ach): Low affinity
- Histaminergic (H1): Low affinity
- Adrenergic (α1): Low affinity

Pharmacokinetics of fluoxetine

Pharmacokinetics: **Non-linear pharmacokinetics**. Fluoxetine has been shown to decrease its own metabolism by the inhibition of the liver enzymes cytochrome P450 2D6 which is the main enzyme responsible for fluoxetine metabolism.

Peak plasma level (Tmax): 6-8 hours

Absorption: Fluoxetine is rapidly absorbed through the intestine, and it is not altered by the presence or absence of food in the stomach. Although food may delay its absorption by 1-2 hours, it does not have any clinical implication.

Steady state: 4 weeks.

Protein binding: **94.5%** mostly to albumin and to α1glycoprotein.

Half-life (t ½):   **Fluoxetine 2-4 days;**
                         Norfluoxetine 7 – 15 days

Bioavailability 72%

Metabolism: CYP 450 enzymes: : **2D6**
Fluoxetine's principal metabolite, *norfluoxetine*, is three times more selective for SERT than the parent drug.

Elimination: Urine 80%
                 Faeces 20%

How supplied

- Tablet 10 mg,
- Capsules 10mg, 20 mg, 40 mg
- Liquid 20mg/5ml bottles and 120 ml bottles

Dose range

- 20 mg – 80 mg for depression
- Doses of 60 – 80 mg a day may be required for OCD and Bulimia.

Clinical indications

- Major depression
- Panic disorder
- Obsessive compulsive disorder
- Premenstrual dysphoric syndrome
- Bulimia

How to treat with fluoxetine

- **For Major Depression (MDD)**: Start with 20 mg a day in a single morning dose to be increased up to a maximum of 80mg a day. Activation-related symptoms may develop at the beginning of the treatment with fluoxetine, and consists of elevated energy, increased anxiety and irritability.

How to stop treatment

Due to its long half-life, there is no need for a slow tapering of fluoxetine in order to avoid withdrawal symptoms.

Side effects

Nervous system
- Insomnia
- Agitation, restlessness, jitteriness
- Akathisia
- Tremor, worsening motor symptoms of Parkinson's disease
- Increased sweating
- Flushing
- Headache
- Dizziness
- Seizures
- Mental slowing
- Reduced attention
- Apathy
- Emotional blunting
- Rash

Gastro intestinal
The gastro intestinal side effects can develop within 30 minutes of drug ingestion and are more likely the result of the direct effect of fluoxetine on the intestinal mucosa rather than of its plasma peak levels.

- Decreased appetite
- Nausea,
- vomiting
- dry mouth
- Diarrhea
- constipation
- Possible weight loss

Sexual

- Decreased sex drive
- Delayed ejaculation
- Impotence
- Inability to reach an orgasm

Suicide

The FDA requires all antidepressants to carry a black box warning stating that antidepressant may increase the risk for suicide in persons under the age of 25 years. This warning is based on data suggesting that suicidal ideations and behavior has a 2 fold increase in children and in adolescents, and a 1.5 – fold increase in the 18 – 24 age group.

Fluoxetine side effects that requires immediate attention
- Confusion
- Excitation
- Onset of seizure
- Yellow skin / eyes

- Severe allergic reaction
- Irregular heart beats

Use during pregnancy: FDA risk category C (i.e.: some animal studies showed adverse effects but there are no controlled studies in humans). The use of fluoxetine in the last trimester of pregnancy may be associated with a higher incidence of respiratory distress and pulmonary hypertension, cyanosis, apnea, seizures, temperature instability, vomiting, hypoglycemia, hypotonia, hyperreflexia, tremor, irritability, constant crying and jitteriness, which may require prolonged hospitalization, tube feeding and respiratory support.

Use during lactation: Fluoxetine secreted in the breast milk. Due to its unknown effects on the new born's normal growth and development, breast feeding should be avoided. Assessing the risk versus benefits must be discussed with the patient.

Avoid using fluoxetine in the following cases

- History of seizure
- Prostate hypertrophy
- Proven allergy to fluoxetine

Fluoxetine drug interactions

- **Drug interactions with Warfarin: Increased** risk for risk of bleeding.

- **Drug interaction with protease inhibitors:** Serotonin syndrome.
- **Drug interaction with LSD: Seizure.**
- **Drug interactions with MAOIs**: CNS toxicity-serotonin syndrome.
- **Drug interactions with Beta Blocker**: Increase beta blockers plasma levels.
- **Drug interactions with sildenafil:** Hypotension.
- **Drug interactions with narcotics: Decreased analgesic** effects.
- **Drug interactions with triptans:** Serotonin-syndrome.
- **Drug interactions with lithium:** Serotonin syndrome.
- **Drug interactions with clozapine & Haloperidol:** Increases their blood levels.
- **Drug interaction with Carbamazepine:** Increase carbamazepine blood levels.

Warnings for Fluoxetine

- **Pregnancy: Risk category C**

- **Fluoxetine may cause an increase in suicidal risk in young adults.** The use of antidepressants may increase the risk of suicidal thinking and behavior in children, adolescents and young adults aged 18-24.

- **Serotonin syndrome:** Symptoms may include agitation, dizziness, hallucinations, delirium, seizures and coma along with autonomic instability that includes tachycardia, fluctuating blood pressure, flushing, hyperthermia, tremor, muscular rigidity, myoclonus, hyperreflexia, incoordination.
- **Activation of hypomania or mania:** may occur in 0.1% of fluoxetine treated bipolar patients.
- **Seizure:** May occur in 0.1% of fluoxetine treated patients.
- **Bleeding**: Fluoxetine may increase the risk of bleeding especially whenever it is used with aspirin, warfarin and non-steroidal anti–inflammatory (NSAIDs) drugs.
- **Hyponatremia:** May develop subsequent to the use of fluoxetine, especially in volume depleted patients and in patients on diuretics.
- **Mydriasis:** Fluoxetine should be avoided in patients having uncontrolled narrow-angle glaucoma.
- **Weight loss & altered appetite**: Fluoxetine was associated with anorexia in 11% of treated patients, while 1.4% of the patients reported weight loss.
- ➢ **Renal impairment**: Fluoxetine require reduced dose in mild to moderate renal impairment.

- **Alcohol:** Fluoxetine is not recommended in patients abusing alcohol.
- **MAOI:** Combination of fluoxetine with MAOI may be fatal. Fluoxetine requires 7 day washout period before starting with MAOI. Fluoxetine requires 3 week washout period after MAOI was stopped.
- **Liver impairment**: In patients with dysfunctional livers, doses of fluoxetine should be lowered in order to prevent drug accumulation in the plasma.

Fluoxetine overdose

Fluoxetine is **relatively safe in mono-therapy overdose. A**s a general rule, the bigger the amount of fluoxetine ingested, the worse the reaction will get and the higher the possibility for lethal results. However, the concomitant use of fluoxetine with alcohol and/or with other central nervous depressants such as painkillers or benzodiazepines may result in death cause by respiratory depression.

Overdose symptoms

The most common symptoms of fluoxetine over dose are:
- nausea
- vomiting
- over sedation
- somnolence

- agitation
- abnormal heart rhythm: sinus tachycardia
- QTc prolongation
- dizziness
- sweating
- tremor
- convulsions
- amnesia
- confusion
- seizures
- cyanosis
- rabdomyolysis
- coma

How to manage fluoxetine's overdosed patients: In general, there is no antidote for fluoxetine overdose and the management is mainly supportive, aimed to maintaining respiration, pulse and blood pressure. In the event of a recent overdose with fluoxetine, a stomach washout, possibly with activated charcoal, may help to eliminate the un- absorbed drug and is done with large–bore oro-gastric tube, maintaining appropriate airway protection. In most cases fluoxetine overdose, requires to hospitalize the patient for at least 24 hours for intense observation.

Fluoxetine references

1 Emslie G.J., Heiligenstein J., Wagner K.D , et al. Fluoxetine for acute treatment of depression in children and adolescent. J. of the American academy of child and adolescent psychiatry. 2002; 41, 1205-1215.

2 Becch P., Cialdella P, Haungh M, et al. Meta analysis of randomized controlled trials of fluoxetine versus placebo and TCA in the short term of MDD. J. of Psychiatry. 2000;176: 421-428.

3 Mcgareth PJ, Stewart J, Quitkin F, et al. Predictors of relapse in a prospective study of fluoxetine treatment of MDD. Am. J. Psychiatry 2006;163: 1542-1548.

4 Michelson D, Allgolacher C, Danlofer K et al. Efficacy of usual antidepressant regims of fluoxetine in panic disorder. B. J. of psychiatry 2001;179: 514-518.

Eight
Fluvoxamine

Brand name: Luvox

Mode of action

- Fluvoxamine is a Serotonin Reuptake Transporter (SERT): Antagonist.
- Fluoxetine is a Sigma 1 receptors agonist.
- Anticholinergic (Ach): Low affinity
- Histaminergic (H1):   Low affinity
- Adrenergic (α1):   Low affinity

Pharmacokinetics of clomipramine

Pharmacokinetics: **Non-linear pharmacokinetics**. Each dose increase of fluvoxamine leads to a disproportionate increase in fluvoxamine plasma levels.

Peak plasma level (T_{max}): 3-8 hours

Absorption: Fluvoxamine is well absorbed by the gastrointestinal system and its absorption is *not affected* by the presence of food.

Steady state: 7 days.

Protein binding: 80% mostly to albumin.

Half-life (t ½): 15 hours

Bioavailability 53%

Metabolism: CYP 450 enzymes: **3A4, 1A2, 2C9** and **2C19**
Fluvoxamine has several **inactive metabolites**.

Elimination: Urine 94%
                    Faeces 6%

How supplied

- Tablet: 25mg, 50mg, 100mg,
- Controlled released tablets (CR): 100mg and 150mg

Dose range

- 100 mg – 200 mg for depression
- 100mg – 300mg for OCD
- 100mg – 300mg for Social anxiety disorder.

Clinical indications (outside the US)

- Depression
- Obsessive compulsive disorder
- Social anxiety disorder
- Post Traumatic Stress Disorder
- Generalised anxiety disorder
- Panic disorder

How to treat with fluvoxamine

- **For Major Depression (MDD)**: Start with 50mg a day in a single morning dose. Wait at least one week to assess clinical improvement before increasing the dose in increments of 50mg a day to a maximum of 200mg a day. With the CR formulation, start with initial dose of 100mg a day to be increased by 50 mg/day weekly up to a maximum of 200mg/day, if needed.

- **For OCD**: Start with 50mg a day to be increased weekly up to a maximum of 300mg a day if required.

- **For Panic disorder, Social anxiety and PMDD**: as for depression.

As a general rule, the higher the patient's anxiety is, the lower the starting dose should be and the slower the dose increase should be in order to minimize the risk of activation.

How to stop treatment

Due to its short half-life, and the potential to develop withdrawal syndrome, a slow tapering of fluvoxamine is highly recommended.

Fluvoxamine discontinuation reaction

The most common symptoms of sudden discontinuation of fluvoxamine are:

- Nausea
- Stomach cramps
- Sweating
- tingling
- dizziness
- light-handedness
- vertigo
- feeling of electricity in the body
- anxiety

Side effects

Nervous system

- Agitation
- Restlessness
- Jitteriness
- anxiety
- Tremor
- increased sweating
- flushing
- headache
- dizziness
- seizures (rare)
- somnolence
- cognitive slowing
- reduced attention
- apathy
- emotional blunting
- rash

Gastro intestinal (GI)

The gastro intestinal side effects can develop within 30 minutes of drug ingestion, and they are more likely the result of the direct effect of fluvoxamine on the intestinal mucosa than the plasma peak level.

- decreased appetite
- upper gastrointestinal symptoms
- nausea

- vomiting
- dry mouth
- diarrhea
- constipation
- Possible weight loss

Sexual

The incidence of the sexual side effects attributed to all the SSRIs is approximately between 20% - 40% of treated patients.

The sexual side effects of fluvoxamine are dose-dependent and do not diminish over time.

The most common fluvoxamine sexual side effects are:

- decreased sex drive
- delayed ejaculation
- impotence
- Inability to reach an orgasm

Suicide

The FDA requires all antidepressants to carry a black box warning stating that antidepressant may increase the risk for suicide in persons under the age of 25 years. This warning is based on data suggesting that suicidal ideations and behavior has a 2 fold increase in children and in adolescents, and a 1.5 – fold increase in the 18 – 24 age group.

Fluvoxamine side effects that requires immediate attention

- Confusion
- Excitation
- Onset of seizure
- Yellow skin / yellow eyes
- Severe allergic reaction
- Irregular heart beats
- Low blood pressure
- Bruising and bleeding(relatively rare)
- Induction of manic episode
- Activation of suicidal ideation and behaviour

Use during pregnancy: FDA risk category C (i.e.: some animal studies showed adverse effects but there are no controlled studies in humans). The use of fluvoxamine in the last trimester of pregnancy may be associated with a higher incidence of respiratory distress and pulmonary hypertension, cyanosis, apnea, seizures, temperature instability, vomiting, hypoglycemia, hypotonia, hyperreflexia, tremor, irritability, constant crying and jitteriness, which may require prolonged hospitalization, tube feeding and respiratory support.

Use during lactation: Fluvoxamine is secreted in the breast milk. Due to its unknown effects on the new born's normal growth and development, breast feeding should be avoided.

Avoid using fluoxetine in the following cases

- History of seizure
- Prostate hypertrophy
- Proven allergy to duloxetine

Fluvoxamine drug interactions

- **Drug interactions with Warfarin: Increased** risk for risk of bleeding.
- **Drug interaction with Buspirone:** 3-fold increase in buspirone plasma levels.
- **Drug interaction with Carbamazepine:** Increase carbamazepine blood levels.
- **Drug interactions with MAOIs:** CNS toxicity-serotonin syndrome.
- **Drug interactions with Statines:** Increase statins blood levels.
- **Drug interactions with Caffeine & Teophilline:** Increase caffeine& Teophilline blood levels.
- **Drug interactions with Alprazola & triazolam:** Increase their blood levels.
- **Drug interactions with propranolol & metoprolol** : Increased propranolol & metoprolol blood levels 5–fold.
- **Drug interactions with Tramadol:** Seizures.

- **Drug interactions with sildenafil:** Increase sildenafil blood levels.
- **Drug interaction with Methadone:** Increase methadone blood levels.

Warnings for Fluvoxamine

- **Pregnancy: Risk category C**

- **Fluvoxamine may cause an increase in suicidal risk in young adults.** The use of antidepressants may increase the risk of suicidal thinking and behavior in children, adolescents and young adults aged 18-24.
- **Serotonin syndrome:** Symptoms may include agitation, dizziness, hallucinations, delirium, seizures and coma along with autonomic instability that includes tachycardia, fluctuating blood pressure, flushing, hyperthermia, tremor, muscular rigidity, myoclonus, hyperreflexia, incoordination.
- **Activation of hypomania or mania:** may occur in 1% of fluvoxamine treated bipolar patients.
- **Seizure:** May occur in 0.2% of fluvoxamine treated patients.
- **Bleeding**: Fluvoxamine may increase the risk of bleeding especially whenever it is used with aspirin, warfarin and non-steroidal anti–inflammatory (NSAIDs) drugs.

- **Hyponatremia:** May develop subsequent to the use of fluvoxamine, especially in volume depleted patients and in patients on diuretics.
- **Mydriasis:** Fluvoxamine should be avoided in patients having uncontrolled narrow-angle glaucoma.
- ➢ **Liver dysfunction.** Fluvoxamine requires dose reduction in patients with liver dysfunction due to its extensive metabolism by the liver CYP 450 enzymatic system
- ➢ **Renal impairment:** Fluvoxaminee require reduced dose in mild to moderate renal impairment.
- **Alcohol:** Fluvoxamine is not recommended in patients abusing alcohol.
- **MAOI:** Combination of fluvoxamine with MAOI may be fatal. Fluvoxamine requires 7 day washout period before starting with MAOI. Fluvoxamine requires 3 week washout period after MAOI was stopped.
- **Elderly.** Fluvoxamine requires lower dose in the elderly due to a longer half-life in patients above 65 years.

Fluvoxamine overdose

Although fluvoxamine **is relatively safe** and **rarely lethal in mono therapy overdose,** a combination of fluvoxamine with alcohol and/ or with other central nervous system depressants such as painkillers or benzo-diazepines may result in death cause by respiratory and cardiovascular depression.

Overdose symptoms

The most common symptoms of fluoxetine over dose are:

- vomiting
- over sedation
- somnolence
- agitation
- dizziness
- diarrhea
- abnormal heart rhythm
- tachycardia
- bradycardia
- hypokalemia
- hypotension
- nausea
- respiratory difficulties
- tremor
- convulsion
- coma

How to manage fluvoxamine's overdosed patients

In general, there is no antidote for fluvoxamine overdose and the management is mainly supportive, aimed to maintaining respiration, pulse and blood pressure. In the event of a recent overdose with fluvoxamine, a stomach washout, possibly with activated charcoal, may help to eliminate the un-absorbed drug and is done with large–bore oro-gastric tube, maintaining appropriate airway protection. In most cases fluvoxamine overdose, requires to hospitalize the patient for at least 24 hours for intense observation.

Fluvoxamine reference

1 Ther P, . The pharmacology of sigma – 1 receptors. Pharmacol Ther, November 2009; 124(2): 195-206.

2 Yasui- Furukori N, Takahta T, Nakaguri T. Different inhibitory effects of fluvoxamine on omeprazole . Br. J. Clin. Pharmacology, April 2004;57 (4) 487 – 494.

3 Dalery J, Honing A. Fluvoxamine versus Fluoxetine in MDD: A double-blind randomised comparison. Human Psychopharmacol Clin Exp 2003: 18:379-384.

4 Figgit DP, McClellan KJ,. Fluvoxamine: an update review of its use in the management of adults with anxiety disorders. Drugs, 2000; 60(4): 925-954.

5 Ravizza L, Barzega G, Bellino S. Drug treatment of obsessive-compulsive disorder (OCD): long-term trial with clomipramine and selective serotonin reuptake inhibitors (SSRIs)Psychopharmacol Bull. 1996;32:167–73.

6 Martin AJ, Wakelin J,. Fluvoxamine: a baseline study of clinical response, long term tolerance and safety in a general practice population. Br J Clin Pract 40-:95-99, 1986.

7 Freeman CP, Trimble MR, Deakin JFW et al: Fluvoxamine versus clomipramine in the treatment of OCD: a multicentre, randomized, double –blind, paralled group cpmparison. J Clin Psychiatry 1994;55(7): 301-305.

Nine

Imipramine

Brand name: Tofranil
Deprinol
Depsonil
Dynaprin
Imipramil

Mode of action

- Imipramine is a potent Serotonin Reuptake Transporter (SERT) antagonist.
- Desipramine (Imipramine's active metabolite) is a potent antagonist of the

Norepinephrine Reuptake Transporter (NET).

- Anticholinergic (Ach): High affinity
- Histaminergic (H1): High affinity
- Adrenergic (α1): High affinity

Pharmacokinetics of imipramine

Pharmacokinetics: **linear pharmacokinetics**. Thus any dose change leads to a proportional change in the drug plasma levels. It appears that there is a relationship between imipramine plasma level and clinical response. Imipramine plasma levels >200ng/mL result in increased efficacy.

Peak plasma level (Tmax): 2-8 hours

Absorption: Imipramine is well absorbed by the gastrointestinal system, mainly in the small intestine. It is not affected by the presence of food.

Steady state: 5-7 days.

Protein binding: **98%** mostly to albumin and to α1-glycoprotein.

Half-life (t ½): 5-30 hours

Bioavailability: Unknown

Metabolism: CYP 450 enzymes: **2D6 and 1A2**
The active metabolite of imipramine is called *desipramine* which has a strong affinity for the presynaptic Norepinephrine Reuptake Transporters (NET).

Elimination: **Urine >80%**

How supplied

- Capsules of 75mg, 125mg, 150mg
- Tablets 10mg, 25mg, 50 mg

Dose range

- Imipramine 50mg -300mg a day for depression

Clinical indications (outside the US)

- Major depression
- Enuresis (involuntary nightly urination during sleep) in children and adolescents.
- Anxiety
- Neuropathic pain
- Insomnia
- Treatment resistant depression
- Cataplexy syndrome

How to treat with imipramine

For Major Depression (MDD): start imipramine with 25mg preferably at bedtime and slowly increase the dose by increments of 25mg every 3 days to a maximum of 300mg taken at bedtime in order to avoid daily sedation. Preferably take imipramine at bedtime to avoid over sedation. In general, "start low and go slow", as patients can experience over-sedation the following day at the beginning of the treatment.

How to stop treatment

It is highly recommended to slow taper imipramine in order to minimize the emergence of withdrawal symptoms, which usually develop within the first 2 weeks of treatment cessation. Imipramine requires a gradual dose reduction in order to avoid discontinuation symptoms.

Imipramine discontinuation reaction

The most common symptoms of sudden discontinuation of imipramine are:

- irritability
- agitation
- dizziness
- anxiety
- confusion

- headache
- lethargy
- insomnia
- seizures
- dysphoric mood
- fever
- fatigue
- sweating
- myalgia (muscle pain)

Side effects

Nervous system
- numbness
- paresthesis of extremities
- incoordination
- ataxia
- extrapyramidal symptoms
- drowsiness
- lethargy
- fatigue
- weakness
- dizziness
- insomnia
- nausea
- blurred vision
- headache and worsening of migraine
- in coordination
- tremor

- disturbed concentration
- disorientation
- confusion
- restlessness and agitation (rare)
- *seizures*.
- stuttering
- disturbance in gait
- worsening of parkinsonism
- rush (rare)
- hypotension
- syncope
- bradycardia

Gastro intestinal
The gastro intestinal side effects can develop within 30 minutes of drug ingestion, and they are more likely the result of imipramine's effects on serotonin uptake and its anticholinergic effects.

- *decreased appetite*
- *heartburn*
- **weight gain (up to 18% of treated patients)**
- nausea
- vomiting
- dry mouth
- constipation
- gastritis
- diarrhea

- peculiar taste
- black tongue
- stomatitis
- abdominal cramps
- epigastric distress
- anorexia

Sexual
- decreased libido
- impotence
- retrograde ejaculation
- painful ejaculation
- delayed ejaculation

Endocrine
- gynecomastia in males
- galactorrhea in female
- breast enlargement in females
- testicular swelling
- Syndrome of inappropriate antidiuretic hormone (SIADH).

Hematologic
- thrombocytopenia
- purpura
- eosinophilia
- agranulocytosis

Allergic
- skin rash
- urticarial

- itching
- photosensitization
- edema
- cross sensitivity with desipramine

Suicide

The FDA requires all antidepressants to carry a black box warning stating that antidepressant may increase the risk for suicide in persons under the age of 25 years. This warning is based on data suggesting that suicidal ideations and behavior has a 2 fold increase in children and in adolescents, and a 1.5 – fold increase in the 18 – 24 age group.

Imipramine side effects that requires immediate attention

- Confusion
- Excitation
- Onset of seizure
- Yellow skin / eyes
- Severe allergic reaction
- Irregular heart beats
- Hypotension
- Induction of manic or hypomanic episode
- Activation of suicidal ideation and behaviour especially in children and adolescents

Use during pregnancy: FDA risk category D (i.e. positive evidence of risk to human fetus however, there have been no well – controlled studies with pregnant women). The use of imipramine in the last trimester of pregnancy may be associated with a higher incidence of respiratory distress and pulmonary hypertension, cyanosis, apnea, seizures, temperature instability, vomiting, hypoglycemia, hypotonia, hyperreflexia, tremor, irritability, constant crying and jitteriness, which may require prolonged hospitalization, tube feeding and respiratory support.

Use during lactation: Imipramine is secreted in the breast milk. Due to its unknown effects on the new born's normal growth and development, breast feeding should be avoided.

Avoid using imipramine in the following cases

- **Hyperthyroidism** Patients with hyperthyroidism are more sensitive to imipramine's side effects.
- **Cardiac arrhythmia**: Patients with pre-existing cardiac disease and cardiac arrhythmias should be closely monitored and preferably avoid the use of imipramine.
- **Mycardial infarction**
- **History of seizure**
- **Prostate hypertrophy**
- **Pre-existing closed angle glaucoma due to imipramine's anticholinergic effects.**

- Proven allergy to imipramine.

Imipramine drug interactions

- **Drug interactions with Warfarin: Increased** PT time and risk for bleeding.
- **Drug interaction with Tramadol:** Seizure.
- **Drug interaction with Carbamazepine:** Decrease imipramine blood levels.
- **Drug interactions with MAOIs:** CNS toxicity-serotonin syndrome.
- **Drug interactions with Akineton:** Increase risk for anticholinergic effects.
- **Drug interactions with Fluoxetine, Fluvoxamine, Paroxetine, Duloxetine, Bupropion, Methylphenidate, Cimetidine, Ketoconazole:** Increase imipramine blood levels.
- **Drug interactions with Phebnobarbital:** Increase phenobarbital blood levels.
- **Drug interactions with Antiarrhytmic:** Prolongs cardiac conduction.
- **Drug interactions with Tamoxifen:** Decrease imipramine blood levels.
- **Drug interactions with Triptans:** Serotonin syndrome.

Warnings for Imipramine

- **Pregnancy: Risk category D**

- **Imipramine may cause an increase in suicidal risk in young adults.** The use of antidepressants may increase the risk of suicidal thinking and behavior in children, adolescents and young adults aged 18-24.

- **Serotonin syndrome:** Symptoms may include agitation, dizziness, hallucinations, delirium, seizures and coma along with autonomic instability that includes tachycardia, fluctuating blood pressure, flushing, hyperthermia, tremor, muscular rigidity, myoclonus, hyperreflexia, incoordination.

- **Activation of hypomania or mania:** may occur in imipramine treated bipolar patients.

- **Seizure:** Imipramine doses higher than 300mg are associated with increased risk of seizure.

- **Cardiac impairment:** Imipramine needs to be used with caution in patients with cardiac impairment. Imipramine use was associated with low blood pressure, ECG abnormalities including ST-T wave changes, PVCs and intraventricular conduction abnormalities. An ECG should be recorded prior to treatment initiation with imipramine.

- **S/P MI:** Imipramine should be avoided in patients who recently had a myocardial infarct.

- **Urinary retention**: Imipramine may worsen urinary retention in predisposed patients due to its anticholinergic properties.
- **Hyperthyroidism:** Imipramine's cardiac toxicity may be increased in patients with hyperthyroidism or patients on thyroid medications.
- **Adrenal medulla tumors:** Imipramine use in patients with adrenal tumors such as pheochromocytoma or neuroblastoma may be associated with hypertensive crisis.
- **Hematologic changes**: Imipramine may be associated with leukopenia, agranulocytosis, thrombocytopenia, anemia, and pancytopenia. Leukocyte and a differential blood count should be obtained immediately in patients who develop fever and sore throat.
- **Hyperthermia**: Imipramine may be associated with hyperthermia, especially when it was used in combination with other drugs.
- **ECT**: The concurrent use of imipramine with ECT may increase the cardiac related hazards of ECT.
- **Mydriasis:** Imipramine should be avoided in patients having uncontrolled narrow-angle glaucoma.
- ➤ **Liver dysfunction**. Imipramine must be avoided in patients with liver dysfunction

due to its extensive metabolism by the liver CYP 450 enzymatic system.

- ➢ **Renal impairment**: Imipramine require reduced dose in mild to moderate renal impairment.
- **Alcohol:** Imipramine is not recommended in patients abusing alcohol.
- **MAOI:** Combination of fluvoxamine with MAOI may be fatal. Fluvoxamine requires 7 day washout period before starting with MAOI. Fluvoxamine requires 3 week washout period after MAOI was stopped.
- **Elderly:** Imipramine requires lower dose in the elderly. Elderly patients with cardiac disease are at special risk of developing cardiac abnormalities.

Imipramine overdose

Imipramine may be lethal in mono therapy overdose as it has a high incidence of fatalities. In addition, the concomitant use of imipramine with alcohol and with other central nervous system depressants such as painkillers or benzo-diazepines may result in death caused by respiratory depression. The possible fatalities are often the result of cardio-respiratory arrest, or with the metabolic acidosis and hypoxia associated with status epilepticus.

Overdose symptoms

The most common symptoms of imipramine over dose are:

- over sedation
- drowsiness
- respiratory depression
- cyanosis
- respiratory arrest
- seizure
- abnormal heart rhythm – mainly tachycardia
- ECG changes – in QRS axis
- congestive heart failure
- cardiac arrest
- hypotension
- hyperactive reflexes
- muscle rigidity
- coreiform movements
- mydriasis
- oliguria
- anuria
- vomiting
- delirium
- disorientation
- hallucinations
- delusions
- anxiety
- restlessness
- agitation

- loss of consciousness

How to manage imipramine's overdosed patients: In general, there is no antidote for imipramine overdose and the management is mainly supportive, aimed to maintaining respiration, pulse and blood pressure. In the event of a recent overdose with imipramine, a stomach washout, possibly with activated charcoal, may help to eliminate the un-absorbed drug and is done with large–bore oro-gastric tube, maintaining appropriate airway protection. In most cases imipramine overdose, requires to hospitalize the patient for at least 24 hours for intense observation.

Imipramine references

1 Avanti A, Kulhare P, Singh G, et al. Comparison of the efficacy and safety of moclobemide and imipramine in the treatment of depression in Indian patients. India J of Psychiatry. 2005 47(2) 84-88.

2 Preskon SH, Irwin HA. Toxicity of TCA: kinetics, mechanism, intervention. J Clin Psychiatry 1982:43:151-156.

3 Bock J, Nelson JC, Gray S et al. Desipramine hydroxylation: variability and effect of antidepressant drugs. Clin Pharmacol Ther , 1983, 33: 190-197.

7 Frank E, Kupfer DJ, Perel JM, et al. Three – years outcome for maintenance therapies in recurrent depression. Arch Gen Psychiatry, 1990, 47:1093-1099.

Ten
Milnacipran

- **Brand name**:
- Toledomin
- Savella
- Ixel
- Dalcipran

Mode of action

- **Milnacipran is a potent Serotonin Reuptake Transporter (SERT): Antagonist.**
- **Milnacipran is a Norepinephrine Reuptake Transporter (NET): Antagonist**
- **Milnacipran increases dopamine levels in the prefrontal cortex by inhibition of the prefrontal (NET).**
- **At higher doses, milnacipran antagonises the NMDA receptors.**

- **Anticholinergic (Ach)**   **Low affinity**
- **Histaminergic (H1):**   **Low affinity**
- **Adrenergic (α1):**   **Lowaffinity**

Pharmacokinetics of milnacipran

Pharmacokinetics: **linear pharmacokinetics**. Thus any dose change leads to a proportional change in the drug plasma levels.

Peak plasma level (T_{max}): 2 hours

Absorption: Milnacipran is well absorbed by the gastrointestinal system, and it is not affected by the presence of food. After oral administration, milnacipran Cmax is reached within 2-4 hours.

Steady state: 36-48 hours.

Protein binding: **13%** mostly to albumin and to α1-glycoprotein.

Half-life ($t \frac{1}{2}$): 8 hours

Bioavailability: 85%

Metabolism: CYP 450 enzymes: **3A4**

Elimination: Urine 90%
                Faeces 10%

How supplied

- Capsule 25mg, 50mg, 100mg

Dose range

- 100 mg – 200 mg for depression in divided doses
- 200mg for fibromyalgia in divided doses.

Clinical indications

- Major depression
- Fibromyalgia
- Chronic muscular pain

How to treat with milnacipran

- **For major depression (MDD)**: start with 25 mg twice a day to be increased up to a maximum of 200mg a day.

- **For fibromyalgia and neuropathic pain**: start with 25 mg twice a day to be increased gradually up to a maximum of 200 mg a day. Doses above 200mg were not associated with a better efficacy.

Milnacipran should be taken in two divided doses. Patients must avoid crushing or chewing the capsule as it will interfere with the drug absorption.

How to stop treatment

Due to its relatively short half-life, there is a need for a slow tapering of milnacipran in order to avoid withdrawal symptoms. In the event of the patient getting withdrawal symptoms, re-instate the previous dose, and once the symptoms disappear, reduce the milnacipran dose in lower proportions and over a longer period of time.

Milnacipran discontinuation reaction

The most common symptoms of sudden discontinuation of milnacipran are:

- Irritability
- Agitation
- Dizziness
- Electric shock sensations
- Anxiety
- Confusion
- Headache
- Lethargy
- Insomnia
- Seizures
- Dysphoric mood

Side effects

Nervous system: The activation syndrome is less common for milnacipran. Common neurological side effects include:

- Insomnia
- Restlessness,
- Restless leg syndrome,
- Muscle spasm
- Tremor
- Hot flashes
- Headache
- Dizziness
- Seizures (rare, mainly associated with treatment discontinuation)
- Increased sweating
- Fatigue
- Somnolence
- Rash

Gastro-intestinal

The GI symptoms are quite common with milnacipran and usually develop within 30 minutes of drug ingestion. The GI side effects are more likely the result of the direct effect of milnacipran on the intestinal mucosa tather than the plasma peak level. The most common GI side effects of milnacipran include:

- Decreased appetite
- Nausea
- Vomiting

- Dry mouth
- Diarrhea
- Constipation
- Possible weight loss
- Gastritis 1%
- Blood in the stools

Anticholinergic

- Dry mouth
- Constipation
- Narrow angle glaucoma
- Dysuria
- Urinary retention
- Urinary hesitancy

Sexual

The sexual side effects of milnacipran are substantial and probably related to its effects on the serotonin levels. They include:

- Decreased sex drive
- Testicular pain
- Testicular swelling
- Delayed ejaculation
- Impotence
- Abnormal orgasm
- Hematuria

Suicide

The FDA requires all antidepressants to carry a black box warning stating that antidepressant may increase the risk for suicide in persons under the age of 25 years. This warning is based on data suggesting that suicidal ideations and behavior has a 2 fold increase in children and in adolescents, and a 1.5 – fold increase in the 18 – 24 age group.

Milnacipran side effects that requires immediate attention

- Confusion
- Excitation
- Onset of seizure
- Yellow skin / eyes
- Severe allergic reaction
- Irregular heart beats
- Hypertension
- Induction of manic or hypomanic episode
- Activation of suicidal ideation and behaviour

Use during pregnancy: FDA risk category C. The use of milnacipran in the last trimester of pregnancy may be associated with a higher incidence of respiratory distress and pulmonary hypertension, cyanosis, apnea, seizures, temperature instability, vomiting, hypoglycemia, hypotonia, hyperreflexia, tremor, irritability, constant crying and jitteriness, which may require prolonged hospitalization, tube feeding and respiratory support.

Use during lactation: Milnacipran is secreted in the breast milk. The maximum estimated daily infant dose of milnacipran from the breast milk was 5% of that of the maternal dose. Due to its unknown effects on the new born's normal growth and development, breast feeding should be avoided.

Avoid using milnacipran in the following cases

- History of seizure
- Prostate hypertrophy
- Pre-existing closed angle glaucoma due to milnaciprane's anticholinergic effects.
- Proven allergy to milnacipran.

Milnacipran drug interactions

- **Drug interactions with Warfarin: Increased** PT time and risk for bleeding.
- **Drug interaction with Tramadol:** Seizure.

- **Drug interaction with Carbamazepine:** Decrease milnacipran blood levels.
- **Drug interactions with MAOIs:** CNS toxicity-serotonin syndrome.
- **Drug interactions with Triptans:** Serotonin syndrome.
- **Drug interactions with Epinephrine:** Hypertensive crisis.

Warnings for milnacipran

- **Pregnancy: Risk category C**

- **Milnacipran may cause an increase in suicidal risk in young adults.** The use of antidepressants may increase the risk of suicidal thinking and behavior in children, adolescents and young adults aged 18-24.
- **Serotonin syndrome:** Symptoms may include agitation, dizziness, hallucinations, delirium, seizures and coma along with autonomic instability that includes tachycardia, fluctuating blood pressure, flushing, hyperthermia, tremor, muscular rigidity, myoclonus, hyperreflexia, incoordination.
- **Activation of hypomania or mania:** may occur in milnacipran treated bipolar patients.
- **Kidney failure:** Milnacipran should be used cautiously in patients with kidney failure.

- **Hypertension:** The effects of Milnacipran on the norepinephrine (NE) system can lead to increased heart rates and blood pressure. Milnacipran was associated with a pulse elevated by 7 beats / minute.

- **Urinary hesitancy:** Milnacipran's ability to potentiate norepinephrine (NE) can increase urethral resistance, which might lead to urinary hesitancy. Male patients with dysuria, benign prostatic hyperplasia and prostatitis may be at higher risk for this side effect.

- **Testicular pain:** Milnacipran was associated with testicular pain and male ejaculation disorders.

- **Seizures:** Although milnacipran use was not associated with increased frequency of seizures, it should be given with care to patients with a history of seizures.

- **Jaundice:** Milnacipran must be discontinued in patients who develop jaundice.

- **Hyponatremia:** Milnacipran use may be associated with hyponatremia, and it is more common in the elderly and in patients taking diuretics. The symptoms of hyponatremia include headache, weakness, reduced concentration, and confusion. In severe cases, hyponatremia can be associated with syncope, hallucinations, seizures and respiratory arrest.

- **Bleeding**: Milnacipran may increase the risk of bleeding events. Thus the concomitant use of aspirin, non-steroidal anti-inflammatory medications and warfarin may increase this risk.
- **Benign prostatic hyperplasia (BPH)**: Milnacipran should be used with caution in patients with BPH due to possible urinary hesitancy and urinary retention.
- **Liver insufficiency**: Milnacipran must be avoided in patients with liver insufficiency.
- **Alcohol abuse**: Milnacipran is not recommended in patients abusing alcohol
- **MAOI**: Milnacipran requires a 2-week washout period before starting with MAOI. A 3-week washout period is required after MAOI was stopped before starting milnacipran.

Milnacipran overdose

Milnacipran **appears to be safe and not lethal in mono therapy overdose**. However, In the concomitant use of milnacipran with alcohol and with other central nervous system depressants such as painkillers or benzo-diazepines may result in death caused by respiratory depression. The possible fatalities are often the result of cardio-respiratory arrest, or with the metabolic acidosis and hypoxia associated with status epilepticus.

Overdose symptoms

The most common symptoms of milnacipran over dose are:
- vomiting
- over sedation/ agitation
- dilated pupils
- abnormal heart rhythm- tachycardia
- hypertension
- cardio respiratory arrest
- confusional state
- dizziness
- increased hepatic enzymes.

How to manage milnaciprane's overdosed patients: In general, there is no antidote for milnacipran overdose and the management is mainly supportive, aimed to maintaining respiration, pulse and blood pressure. In the event of a recent overdose with milnacipran, a stomach washout, possibly with activated charcoal, may help to eliminate the un-absorbed drug and is done with large–bore oro-gastric tube, maintaining appropriate airway protection. In most cases milnacipran overdose, requires to hospitalize the patient for at least 24 hours for intense observation.

Milnacipram references

1 Kasper S, Pletan Y, Solles A et al. Comparative studies with milnacipran and TCA in the treatment of patients with MDD. A summery of clinical trials. Int. Cl. Psych. 1996:11 (Supp. 4): 35-39.

2 Ansseau, A., Ppat P., Troisfotains B.   Controlled Comparrison of milnacipran and fluoxetine in MDD. Psych. 1994:114:131-137.

3 Papakostas G.L, Fava M. A meta- analysis of clinical trials comparing milnacipran, an SNRI, with SSRI for the treatment of MDD. European neuropsychopharmacology, 2007: 20(17), 32 – 36.

4 Rouillon F, Warner B, Pezous N et al. Milnacipran recurrence prevention study group: milnacipram efficacy in the prevention of recurrent depression: a 12-month placebo-controlled study. Int. Clin. Psychopharmacology 2000;15:133-140.

Eleven

Mirtazapine

- **Brand name**: Remeron

Mode of action

- Mirtazapine is an α-2 adrenergic auto-receptor antagonist
- Mirtazapine is a 5-HT2c antagonist
- Mirtazapine is a 5–HT2A antagonist
- Mirtazapine is a 5-HT3 antagonist
- Anticholinergic (Ach)   Low affinity
- Histaminergic (H1):   High affinity
- Adrenergic (α1):   Low affinity

Pharmacokinetics of mirtazapine

Pharmacokinetics: Mirtazapine has **linear pharmacokinetics.** Thus increased doses of mirtazapine result in proportionally increased blood levels.

Peak plasma level (T_{max}): 2 hours

Absorption: Mirtazapine is well absorbed by the gastrointestinal system and **it is not affected by the presence of food in the stomach.**

Steady state: 5-7 Days.

Protein binding: **85%** mostly to albumin and to α1-glycoprotein.

Half-life ($t \frac{1}{2}$): 20-40 hours

Bioavailability: 50%

Metabolism: CYP 450 enzymes: **2D6, 1A2, 3A3/4.** Mirtazapine is metabolized to *desmethyl active metabolites*. However, due to their low plasma concentrations, these active metabolites have marginal clinical effects.

Elimination: Urine 75%
                Faeces 15%
The clearance of mirtazapine can be reduced by 30% – 50% in patients with renal impairment.

How supplied

- Tablets 15mg, 30mg, 45mg.
- Disintegrating tablets called Soltab15,30,45mg which dissolve on the tongue within 30 seconds

Dose range

- 15 – 45 mg once daily at bedtime for the treatment of major depression.

Clinical indications

- Major depression
- Panic disorder
- Generalized anxiety disorder (GAD)
- Post Traumatic Stress Disorder (PTSD)

How to treat with mirtazapine

For depression: start with mirtazapine 15mg at bedtime and increase the dose every 7 days until you reach the desired antidepressant effect. In severe cases, a maximum of 45mg can be given once daily at bedtime.

How to stop treatment

A sudden discontinuation of mirtazapine use can lead to discontinuation syndrome. A slow tapering of mirtazapine is recommended.

Mirtazapine discontinuation reaction

The most common symptoms of sudden discontinuation of mirtazapine are:

- Anxiety
- Irritability
- Agitation
- Dizziness
- Flu like symptoms
- Confusion
- Headache
- Lethargy
- Insomnia
- Seizures
- Dysphoric mood

Side effects

Nervous system
- Sedation- May develop in 30% of patients
- Fatigue
- Insomnia
- Agitation

- Restlessness,
- Muscle pain
- Vivid dreams
- hallucinations
- Headache
- Dizziness
- *Seizures* (very rare)
- Rash
- Dry mouth
- Blurred vision
- Hypotension
- Palpitation
- Vertigo
- Pupil dilatation

Gastro intestinal

GI side effects are less common with mirtazapine. However, increased appetite and weight gain are highly frequent with mirtazapine use.

- **increased appetite**
- **weight gain** – May develop in 17% of patients
- nausea ,
- vomiting
- dry mouth
- constipation

Sexual: In general, the use of mirtazapine is associated with lower incidence of sexual dysfunction. The most common sexual side effects of mirtazapine are:

- Decreased sex drive
- Delayed ejaculation
- Impotence
- Abnormal orgasm

Other side effects

- Urinary retention
- Increased body temperature
- Excessive sweating
- Bone marrow suppression- rare
- Agranulocytosis- rare

Suicide

The FDA requires all antidepressants to carry a black box warning stating that antidepressant may increase the risk for suicide in persons under the age of 25 years. This warning is based on data suggesting that suicidal ideations and behavior has a 2 fold increase in children and in adolescents, and a 1.5 – fold increase in the 18 – 24 age group.

Mirtazapine side effects that requires immediate attention

- Confusion
- Excitation
- Onset of seizure

- Yellow skin / eyes
- Severe allergic reaction
- Irregular heart beats
- Hypertension/ hypotension
- Induction of manic or hypomanic episode
- Activation of suicidal ideation and behaviour

Use during pregnancy: FDA risk category C. The use of mirtazapine in the last trimester of pregnancy may be associated with a higher incidence of respiratory distress and pulmonary hypertension, cyanosis, apnea, seizures, temperature instability, vomiting, hypoglycemia, hypotonia, hyperreflexia, tremor, irritability, constant crying and jitteriness, which may require prolonged hospitalization, tube feeding and respiratory support.

Use during lactation: Mirtazapine is secreted in the breast milk. Due to its unknown effects on the new born's normal growth and development, breast feeding should be avoided.

Avoid using mirtazapine in the following cases

- In patients taking MAOI medication
- In patients with proven allergy to mirtazapine
- In patients with a history of seizure

Mirtazapine drug interactions

- **Drug interactions with Fluvoxamine:** Increase mirtazapine blood levels.
- **Drug interaction with Tramadol:** Seizure.
- **Drug interaction with Carbamazepine:** Decrease mirtazapine blood levels by 60%.
- **Drug interactions with MAOIs:** CNS toxicity-serotonin syndrome.
- **Drug interactions with Venlafaxin:** Serotonin syndrome.
- **Drug interactions with Fluvoxamine:** Increase mirtazapine blood levels by 4-fold.

Warnings for mirtazapine

- **Pregnancy: Risk category C**

- **Mirtazapine may cause an increase in suicidal risk in young adults.** The use of antidepressants may increase the risk of suicidal thinking and behavior in children, adolescents and young adults aged 18-24.
- **Serotonin syndrome:** Symptoms may include agitation, dizziness, hallucinations, delirium, seizures and coma along with autonomic instability that includes tachycardia, fluctuating blood pressure, flushing, hyperthermia, tremor, muscular rigidity, myoclonus, hyperreflexia, incoordination.

- **Activation of hypomania or mania:** may occur in 0.2% of mirtazapine treated bipolar patients.
- **The incidence of seizures** is extremely low with mirtazapine use. In all the US clinical trials only one seizure was reported. However, mirtazapine should be used cautiously in patients with a history of seizures
- **Serotonin syndrome** may develop with mirtazapine use.
- **Cardiac impairment**: Mirtazapine needs to be used with caution in patients with cardiac impairment.
- **Co-administration of mirtazapine with tramadol** may increase seizure risk.
- **Renal impairment**: mirtazapine requires a dose adjustment (lower dose) in mild to moderate renal impairment.
- **Alcohol**: Mirtazapine is not recommended in patients abusing alcohol.
- **Elderly**: Mirtazapine needs a dose adjustment (lower dose) in the elderly
- **MAOI:** Mirtazapine combined with MAOI might be fatal. Mirtazapine requires a **7-day** washout period before starting with MAOI. After stopping a MAOI, a **3-week** washout period is required before starting mirtazapine.

- **Withdrawal reaction**. Mirtazapine may cause withdrawal reaction, prevention of which requires a slow reduction of mirtazapine doses. The onset of withdrawal symptoms is attributed to mirtazapine's short half-life as well as to the lack of active metabolites. The withdrawal symptoms of mirtazapine can develop as early as the second day of the drug's sudden discontinuation and may persist for several days. The most common withdrawal symptoms are nausea, dizziness, insomnia, anxiety, tension and headache.

- **Agranulocytosis**: in clinical trials there were **three** cases of agranulocytosis out of 2796 patients treated with mirtazapine. Thus patients should be observed for signs of sore throat, fever, stomatitis or any other signs of infection, and labs should be checked for low WBC count with any signs of infection.

- **Cholesterol**: Non-fasting cholesterol increased by >20% above the upper normal limits in 15% of the patients treated with mirtazapine as compared to 7% for placebo.

- **Triglycerides**: Non-fasting triglycerides increased to >500mg/dL in 6% of patients treated by mirtazapine as compared to 3% of patients on placebo.

- **Transaminase elevation.** Treatment with mirtazapine caused clinically significant

SGPT elevations >3 times the upper normal limit in 2% of patients. However, the transaminase elevation was not associated with compromised liver function.

- **Increased appetite:** weight gain developed in 17% of the patients treated with mirtazapine as compared to 2% for placebo.
- **Somnolence:** somnolence was reported in 54% of the patients treated with mirtazapine compared to 18% on placebo. Somnolence was associated with treatment discontinuation in 10% of mirtazapine treated patients. In addition, increased somnolence may affect performance in activities which require alertness.

Mirtazapine overdose

Mirtazapine is **relatively safe in mono therapy overdose,** with rare incidence of fatalities. However, the concomitant use of mirtazapine with alcohol and with other central nervous depressants such as painkillers or benzo-diazepines may result in death caused by respiratory depression.

Overdose symptoms

The most common symptoms of mirtazapine over dose are:
- Over-sedation
- drowsiness

- disorientation
- impaired memory
- Seizure
- abnormal heart rhythm
- tachycardia
- hallucinations
- vomiting
- loss of consciousness

How to manage mirtazapine's overdosed patients

In general, there is no antidote for mirtazapine overdose and the management is mainly supportive, aimed to maintaining respiration, pulse and blood pressure. In the event of a recent overdose with mirtazapine, a stomach washout, possibly with activated charcoal, may help to eliminate the un-absorbed drug and is done with large–bore oro-gastric tube, maintaining appropriate airway protection. In most cases mirtazapine overdose, requires to hospitalize the patient for at least 24 hours for intense observation.

Mirtazapine References

1 Szegedi A, Muller MJ, Anghelescu I Early improvement under mirtazapine and paroxetine predicts later stable response and remission with high sensitivity in patients with MDD. J of Clin Psychiatry. 2003; 64 (4):413-420.

2 Thase ME. Effectiveness of antidepressants: comparative remission rates. J Clin Psychiatry 2003: 64(Suppl 2): 3-7.

3 Fawcett J, Barkin RL. Review of the results from clinical studies on the efficacy, safety and tolerability of mirtazapine for the treatment of patients with MDD. J Affective Disorder 1998;51:267-285.

4 Carpenter LL, Yasmin S, Price L. A double blind, placebo controlled study of antidepressant augmentation with mirtazapine. Biol Psychiatry 2002;51:183-188.

5 Guelfi JD, Ansseau M, Timmerman L et al. Mirtazapine versus venlafaxine in hospitalized severely depressed patients with melancholic features. J Clin Psychopharmacol 2001:21:425-431.

6 Freund TF, Gulyas AL. Inhibitory control of GABAergic interneurons in the hippocampus. Can J Physiol Pharmacol. 1997 May; 75(5): 479-87

7 McMahon Lori L, Kauer J.A. Hippocampal Interneurons Express a Novel Form of Synaptic Plasticity. Neouron, February 1997, Vol 18, 295-305.

Twelve

Tranylcypromine

- **Brand name**: Parnate

Mode of action

- Tranylcypromine Irreversible inhibition of MAO–A and MAO–B isoenzymes.
- Anticholinergic (Ach) Moderate affinity
- Histaminergic (H1): Moderate affinity
- Adrenergic (α1): High affinity

Pharmacokinetics of mirtazapine

Pharmacokinetics: Tranylcypromine has **non-linear pharmacokinetics** which implies that any dose-change leads to a dis-proportional change in the drug plasma levels.

Peak plasma level (T_{max}): 1- 2 hours

Absorption: Tranylcypromine is rapidly and well-absorbed by the gastrointestinal system.

Steady state: 5-7 Days.

Protein binding: Highly protein bound, mostly to albumin and to α1-glycoprotein.

Half-life (t ½): 2.5 hours

Bioavailability: 50%

Metabolism: CYP 450 enzymes: **2A6, 2C19 and 2D6**

Elimination: Mostly in the **Urine**.

How supplied

- Tranylcypromine tablets: 10mg

Dose range

- Tranylcypromine 10mg – 60mg a day for the treatment of major depression.

Clinical indications

- Major depression (FDA approved)
- Treatment resistant depression
  Panic disorder

How to treat with mirtazapine

- **For Major Depression (MDD):** start treatment with tranylcypromine 30mg, a day preferably in divided doses. Slowly increase with increments of 10mg a day every seven days up to a maximum of 60mg/day which must be taken also in three divided doses.

Preferably take tranylcypromine in three divided doses of 10mg each in order to minimize the potential development of hypotension and tachycardia. As a general rule, always start with a low dose of 30mg a day and increase in a small proportions over a long period of time.

How to stop treatment

Sudden termination of tranylcypromine use may be associated with the emergence of discontinuation symptoms.
It is highly recommended to reduce the use of tranylcypromine slowly in order to minimize the emergence of withdrawal symptoms, which may develop within 1 – 4 days.

The most recommended option is to reduce the dose of tranylcypromine by 50% every third day. However, in the event of the patient experiencing withdrawal symptoms, re-instate the previous dose of tranylcypromine, and once the discontinuation symptoms disappear, start tapering down the tranylcypromine dose in smaller proportions and over longer period of time.

Tranylcypromine discontinuation reaction

The most common symptoms of sudden discontinuation of tranylcypromine are:

- Irritability
- Agitation
- Dizziness
- Anxiety
- Confusion
- Headache
- Lethargy
- Insomnia
- Seizures
- Dysphoric mood
- Fever
- Fatigue
- Sweating
- Myalgia (muscle pain)
- Hallucinations
- Vivid nightmares

Side effects

Nervous system
- Drowsiness
- Lethargy, fatigue, weakness
- Dizziness
- Sedation
- insomnia
- Headache and worsening of migraine
- Disorientation
- Confusion
- Restlessness and agitation (rare)
- *Seizures* rare
- **Hypotension**
- Syncope
- tachycardia

Anticholinergic effects

- *Decreased appetite*
- *Dry mouth*
- Blurred vision
- Constipation
- Sweating
- Urinary retention

Gastro intestinal side effects: low incidence
- Nausea
- Vomiting

Sexual

- Decreased libido
- Impotence
- Retrograde ejaculation
- Delayed ejaculation

Suicide

The FDA requires all antidepressants to carry a black box warning stating that antidepressant may increase the risk for suicide in persons under the age of 25 years. This warning is based on data suggesting that suicidal ideations and behavior has a 2 fold increase in children and in adolescents, and a 1.5 – fold increase in the 18 – 24 age group.

Tranylcypromine side effects that requires immediate attention

- Confusion
- Excitation
- Onset of seizure
- Yellow skin / eyes
- Severe allergic reaction
- Irregular heart beat
- Hypotension
- Induction of manic or hypomanic episode
- Activation of suicidal ideation and suicidal behaviour especially in children and adolescents under the age of 25 years.

Use during pregnancy: FDA risk category C. The use of tranylcypromine in the last trimester of pregnancy may be associated with a higher incidence of respiratory distress and pulmonary hypertension, cyanosis, apnea, seizures, temperature instability, vomiting, hypoglycemia, hypotonia, hyperreflexia, tremor, irritability, constant crying and jitteriness, which may require prolonged hospitalization, tube feeding and respiratory support.

Use during lactation: Tranylcypromine is secreted in the breast milk. Due to its unknown effects on the new born's normal growth and development, breast feeding should be avoided.

Avoid using tranylcypromine in the following cases

- **Myocardial infarction & cardiac impairment**: Patients who are recovering from myocardial infarction should avoid using tranylcypromine due its propensity to cause hypotension and tachycardia.
- History of seizure
- Liver impairment
- Pheochromocytoma
- Presence of severe headache
- Anorexia & low body weight
- Proven allergy to tranylcypromine
- Co-administration with prohibited medications (see drug interactions)

- Co-administration with food containing high tyramine levels. (See comprehensive list of food and beverages)
- In patients who have a history of drug abuse-especially stimulants

Tranylcypromine drug interactions

- **Drug interaction with all antidepressants:** Serotonin syndrome.
- **Drug interaction with Triptans, ecstasy, Amphetamine, ephedrine, methylphenidate, pseudoephedrine, domapine, tyramine, adrenaline and salbutamol, L- tryptophan :** Serotonin syndrome
- **Drug interactions with Buspiron**: Hypertension.
- **Drug interactions with ACE inhibitors**: Hypotension.
- **Drug interactions with Tramadol:** Seizure.

Hypertensive crisis

Hypertensive crisis is a serious and dangerous medical condition which can develop when patients treated with tranylcypromine will consume a large amount of food that contains high levels of tyramine.

Tyramine is a natural monoamine compound which can be found in food and in plants. Tyramine can also be produced in food and beverages as a result of fermentation and spoilage.

Once ingested, tyramine gets absorbed through the gastro intestinal tract into the blood and distributes all over the body with the exception of the brain as the tyramine molecule is unable to cross the blood-brain barrier. In the human body, tyramine induces the release of dopamine (DA) and norepinephrine (NE) which can cause vasoconstriction and high blood pressure.

In regular circumstances, the MAO–A enzyme, located inside the cells, controls the amount of norepinephrine and dopamine, by the breaking down the excess neurotransmitters.
This normally results in controlled blood pressure.

However, in a patient on tranylcypromine who ingests a large amount of tyramine, the irreversible inhibition of MAO-A enzymes, by MAOI results in a disproportionate increase in norepinephrine and dopamine. This then stimulates the α1 adrenergic receptors in the blood vessel endothelium, causing vasoconstriction and elevated blood pressure.

Food containing tyramine is absorbed through the intestinal wall and gets destroyed immediately by the gastroenteric MAO–A enzymes which act like gate keepers. However, there is always a small amount of tyramine which may escape and leak into the blood stream.

Nevertheless, the second line of defense which protects the body from too much tyramine in the blood is the liver, which is also capable of destroying the free tyramine with its own MAO–A enzymes.

In normal situations, the MAO–A enzyme can handle food containing up to **400mg** of ingested tyramine before any change in blood pressure develops. A high tyramine content meal contains approximately **40mg** of tyramine, which is easily destroyed by the MAO–A enzymes.

However, in the patient on tranylcypromine, the majority of its MAO-A enzyme is inhibited, resulting in limited ability to handle the excess in tyramine, and increasing the patient's vulnerability to develop elevated blood pressures.

Thus, patients on tranylcypromine that consume a meal containing as little as 10mg of tyramine may develop a significant and sudden increase in their blood pressure.

Hypertensive crisis is a surge in blood pressure, which may exceed 180/120mm Hg. Hypertensive crisis is a medical emergency that may cause intracranial bleeding and death.

Hypertensive crisis is divided into two categories: Hypertensive urgency and hypertensive emergency.

> **Hypertensive urgency**: is an acute elevation in blood pressure without end-organ damage.
> **Hypertensive emergency**: is an acute elevation in blood pressure which is accompanied by end-organ damage. Hypertensive emergency can be associated with life-threatening complications such as brain hemorrhage and organs failure.

Causes of hypertensive emergency include

- Poor compliance of blood pressure medications.
- Myocardiac infarction
- Heart failure
- Kidney failure
- Stroke
- Eclampsia
- Food containing high levels of tyramine.

Despite the possible risk of developing hypertensive crisis from foods containing tyramine, tranylcypromine users can still enjoy some foods containing tyramine. For example, one needs to eat more than 20 pieces of pizza or drink the same number of wine or beer glasses before the patient is at risk of developing hypertensive crisis (3).

The physiological effects of incremental tyramine intake in patients using tranylcypromine are as follows:

- ➢ **Tyramine 8mg**: Elevated blood pressure, increased heart rate.
- ➢ **Tyramine 10mg**: Headache, nausea, vomiting.
- ➢ **Tyramine 25mg**: Hypertensive crisis.

The clinical symptoms of hypertensive crisis characterized by the sudden onset of occipital headache, which may radiate frontally, palpitation, neck stiffness, neck pain, nausea, vomiting, sweating, and photophobia. In addition, the patient may experience chest pain, tachycardia and pupil dilation. The cardiac findings of hypertensive crisis include prominent apical pulsation and cardiac enlargement. The funduscopic findings of hypertensive crisis may include papilledema and hemorrhages. Most patients present with blood pressure that exceeds 180/120 mm Hg, which may lead to intracranial bleeding with a fatal outcome.

Hypertensive crisis requires immediate discontinuation of tranylcypromine, as well as therapy to lower blood pressure. These should be given immediately and slowly titrated in order to avoid an excessive drop in blood pressure. Excessive blood pressure lowering should be avoided due to the risk of getting cerebral ischemia if blood pressure falls too quickly.

Oral antihypertensive medication includes:

- ACE inhibitors,
- Beta-blockers
- Calcium channel blocker.

Patient may be observed for several hours and once their blood pressure returns to normal levels they can be followed up as outpatient. Patients with hypertensive emergency should be admitted to an intensive care for close monitoring of hemodynamics, urine output and of other ends-organ damages.

Symptoms of hypertensive crisis are

- Occipital headache,
- Neck stiffness
- Nausea
- Vomiting
- Dilated pupils and photophobia
- Bleeding nose
- Chest pain
- Tachycardia
- Shortness of breath
- Seizures
- Unresponsiveness

Hypertensive crisis is a medical emergency which requires immediate medical intervention with the aim to reduce the elevated blood pressure which may have catastrophic consequences.

Food restrictions when using tranylcypromine

Due to the danger of the serious interactions of tranylcypromine with food containing tyramine, the amount of ingested tyramine must be strictly controlled. Follows a list of food and their tyramine content.

Food containing high levels of tyramine which should be avoided

- All matured aged cheeses: cheddar, blue, Roquefort, camembert
- Marmite
- Broad beans
- Pickled herring & other dried fish
- Soups in packets
- Sauerkraut
- Aged smoked meat
- Beer
- Wine
- Liver
- Hard salami
- Dried sausage
- Pepperoni
- Yogurt
- Tofu

Food containing low tyramine levels which can be ingested in moderation and fresh

- Cottage cheese
- Sour cream
- Salad dressing

As a general rule, fresh food has a low tyramine content, while spoiled and processed food, canned food, gravy sauces and fermented food contain higher levels of tyramine.

Warnings for tranylcypromine

- ➢ **Pregnancy**: **Risk category C**. Try to avoid use during pregnancy or breastfeeding. Assessment of the risks versus benefits must be discussed with the patient.
- ➢ **Tranylcypromine may cause an increase in suicidal risk in young adults**. Tranylcypromine, as all antidepressants used for MDD may increase the risk of suicidal thinking and behavior in children, adolescents and young adults aged 18-24. The use of antidepressants in this population must balance the risk of suicide with the clinical need. Careful monitoring of the patient's clinical worsening, and suicidality should also involve the family and all other caregivers.

➤ **Activation of hypomania or mania** may occur in tranylcypromine treated bipolar patients. As tranylcypromine may trigger mania in predisposed patients, it should be used cautiously in patients with a history of bipolar mood disorder

➤ **Serotonin syndrome** may develop with tranylcypromine use. Symptoms of serotonin syndrome may include agitation, dizziness, hallucinations, delirium, seizures and coma along with autonomic instability including tachycardia, fluctuating blood pressure, flushing, hyperthermia, tremor, muscular rigidity, myoclonus, hyperreflexia, incoordination. The concomitant use of tranylcypromine with antidepressants and triptans may precipitate serotonin syndrome which may be fatal.

➤ **Over-the-counter medications:** Tranylcypromine use combined with many psychotropic and other over the counter medications may cause serotonin syndrome.

➤ **Syncope:** Tranylcypromine use was associated with syncope and hypotension. Postural hypotension may be relieved by having the patient lie down with their legs elevated until blood pressure returns to normal. The concomitant use of tranylcypromine with anti-hypertensive drugs may exacerbate hypotension.

➤ **Heart disease**: Tranylcypromine may have the capacity to suppress angina pain that would otherwise serve as a warning sign for myocardial ischemia. Further, Tranylcypromine is not recommended for use during the initial phase of myocardial infarction as it is associated with QT prolongation and isolated PVCs, tachycardia, syncope and torsades de pointes. Finally, tranylcypromine needs to be used with caution in patients with cardiac impairment and should be avoided in patients who recently had a myocardial infarct.

➤ **Kidney dysfunction.** Tranylcypromine requires a lower dose adjustment in patients with kidney impairment due to its elimination in the urine.

➤ **Liver dysfunction**. Tranylcypromine requires a lower dose adjustment in patients with liver dysfunction due to its extensive metabolism by the liver CYP 450 enzymatic system.

➤ **Elderly:** Tranylcypromine needs a lower dose adjustment in the elderly.

➤ **Seizure:** Tranylcypromine may lower the seizure threshold, thus suitable precautions should be taken in patients with history of seizures..

> ➤ **Alcohol abuse**: Tranylcypromine is not recommended in patients abusing alcohol. In addition, tranylcypromine should be used with caution in patient using disulfiram (antabuse). A study on rats which were given high doses of tranylcypromine plus Antabuse experienced severe toxicity including convulsions and death.

Tranylcypromine overdose

Tranylcypromine **can be lethal in mono therapy overdose,** which may result in a high incidence of fatalities. Moreover, the concomitant use of tranylcypromine with alcohol and/ or with other central nervous depressants such as painkillers or benzo-diazepines may result in death cause by the additive effects of the combined medications on the patient's respiratory system causing respiratory depression and cardio-respiratory arrest, metabolic acidosis and hypoxia.

Overdose symptoms

The most common symptoms of tranylcypromine over dose are:
- over sedation
- respiratory arrest
- seizure
- abnormal heart rhythm – mainly tachycardia
- hypotension

- vomiting
- ataxia
- headache
- restlessness
- confusion
- delirium
- loss of consciousness

How to manage tranylcypromine's overdosed patients: In general, there is no antidote for tranylcypromine overdose and the management is mainly supportive, aimed to maintaining respiration, pulse and blood pressure. In the event of a recent overdose with tranylcypromine, a stomach washout, possibly with activated charcoal, may help to eliminate the un- absorbed drug and is done with large–bore oro-gastric tube, maintaining appropriate airway protection. In most cases tranylcypromine overdose, requires to hospitalize the patient for at least 48 hours for intense observation.

Tranylcypromine references

1 SM Stahl. Stahl's Essential Psychopharmacology, Third edition. Cambridge University Press 2008.

Thirteen

Paroxetine

Brand name: Aropax, Paxil

Mode of action

- Paroxetine is a Serotonin Reuptake Transporter (SERT): Antagonist.
- Paroxetine is a Norepinephrine Reuptake Transporter (NET) antagonist.
- Paroxetin is a Nitric Oxide Synthase (NOS) enzyme inhibitor.
- Anticholinergic (Ach)   Low affinity
- Histaminergic (H1):   Low affinity
- Adrenergic (α1):   Low affinity

Pharmacokinetics of paroxetine

Pharmacokinetics: Paroxetine has **non-linear pharmacokinetics,** and it *inhibits* its own metabolism. Thus, a dose increase of paroxetine may result in a disproportionate increase in paroxetine plasma levels.

Peak plasma level (Tmax):
        6.4 hours– on empty stomach.
        4.9 hours when ingested with food.

Absorption: Paroxetine is rapidly and well-absorbed by the gastrointestinal system.

Steady state: 7-10 Days.

Protein binding: **95%**: mostly to albumin and to α1-glycoprotein.

Half-life (t ½): 21-24 hours

Bioavailability: 100%

Metabolism: CYP 450 enzymes: **2D6**

Paroxetine is metabolized into products conjugated with glucuronic acid and sulphate. These metabolites are clinically inactive.

Elimination: **Urine 65%**
        Faeces 36%

How supplied

- Tablet: 10mg, 20mg, 30mg, 40 mg.
- Controlled released tablets (CR): 12.5mg, 25mg
- Oral solution 10mg/ 5ml

Dose range

- 20 mg – 50 mg for depression

Clinical indications

- Major depression
- Panic disorder
- Obsessive compulsive disorder
- Premenstrual dysphoric disorder
- Post Traumatic Stress Disorder
- Generalised anxiety disorder
  Social anxiety disorder

How to treat with paroxetine

- **For Major Depression (MDD)**: With paroxetine IR start with 20mg a day in a single morning dose. Wait at least two weeks to assess the clinical improvement before increasing the dose to a maximum of 50mg a day.

With paroxetine CR, an initial dose of 25mg a day may be increased by 12.5 mg/day weekly to a maximum of 62.5mg/day.

- **For OCD**: For paroxetine IR start with 20mg a day to be increased weekly by 10 mg up to 60 mg a day if necessary.

- **For Panic disorder (PD), Social anxiety & Post Traumatic Stress disorder (PTSD)**: Start with 10mg a day to avoid excitation and possible anxiety, and increase the dose weekly in increments of 10mg/day to a maximum of 40mg a day. As a general rule, the higher the patient's anxiety, the *lower* the starting dose should be and the *slower* the dose increases.

- **For Premenstrual dysphoric disorder (PMDD)**: Start with paroxetine CR 12.5 mg a day, initiating a week before the menses start. In severe cases take the medicine throughout the menstrual cycle at a maximum dose of 25mg a day.

Patients should take paroxetine preferably in the evening. However, paroxetine can be taken at any time of the day if it is tolerated.

How to stop treatment

Due to its short half-life and the lack of active metabolites paroxetine has a strong potential for withdrawal syndrome, which requires a slow down-titration. The patient need to reduce the dose of paroxetine gradually, with a 50% dose reduction every 3 days.

Paroxetine discontinuation reaction

The most common symptoms of sudden discontinuation of paroxetine are:

- nausea
- insomnia
- dizziness
- light-headedness
- vertigo
- nightmares and vivid dreams
- feelings of electricity in the body
- anxiety

Side effects

Nervous system
- Activation. The activation response is much less common for paroxetine compared to other SSRI medications
- Insomnia
- Agitation,

- Restlessness,
- Jitteriness
- Anxiety
- Tremor,
- Increased sweating
- Flushing
- Headache
- Dizziness
- Seizures (rare)
- Somnolence
- Cognitive slowing
- Reduced attention
- Apathy
- Emotional blunting
- Rash

Gastro intestinal: The GI symptoms are more common with paroxetine and usually develop within 30 minutes of the drug ingestion. They are more likely the result of the direct effect of paroxetine on the intestinal mucosa than to its plasma peak level.

- decreased appetite
- upper gastrointestinal symptoms
- nausea,
- vomiting
- dry mouth
- diarrhoea
- constipation
- possible weight loss

Sexual

The incidence of sexual side effects attributed to the SSRIs is approximately between 20% - 40% of treated patients. The sexual side effects of paroxetine are dose-dependent and do not diminish over time. The most common sexual side effects are:

- Decreased sex drive
- Delayed ejaculation
- Impotence
- Inability to reach an orgasm

Suicide

The FDA requires all antidepressants to carry a black box warning stating that antidepressant may increase the risk for suicide in persons under the age of 25 years. This warning is based on data suggesting that suicidal ideations and behavior has a 2 fold increase in children and in adolescents, and a 1.5 – fold increase in the 18 – 24 age group.

Paroxetine side effects that requires immediate attention

- Confusion
- Excitation
- Onset of seizure
- Yellow skin / eyes
- Severe allergic reaction
- Irregular heart beats
- Low blood pressure
- Bruising and bleeding(relatively rare)

- Induction of manic episode
- Activation of suicidal ideation and behaviour

Use during pregnancy: FDA risk category D. The use of paroxetine in the last trimester of pregnancy may be associated with a higher incidence of respiratory distress and pulmonary hypertension, cyanosis, apnea, seizures, temperature instability, vomiting, hypoglycemia, hypotonia, hyperreflexia, tremor, irritability, constant crying and jitteriness, which may require prolonged hospitalization, tube feeding and respiratory support.

Use during lactation: Paroxetine is secreted in the breast milk. Due to its unknown effects on the new born's normal growth and development, breast feeding should be avoided.

Avoid using paroxetine in the following cases

- Proven allergy to paroxetine
- Co-administration with MAOIs

Paroxetine drug interactions

- **Drug interaction with cimetidine:** Increase paroxetine blood levels.
- **Drug interaction with Tramadol, LSD:** Seizure.
- **Drug interaction with Lithium:** Nausea tremor.
- **Drug interaction with Ritonavir :** Decrease paroxetine blood level.

- **Drug interactions with Pimozide, Thioridazine**: Increase antipsychotics blood levels.
- **Drug interaction with Digoxin:** Decrease digoxin blood levels by 18%.
- **Drug interaction with Phenytoin:** Increase phenithoin blood levels.
- **Drug interactions with Benztropine & Procyclidine**: Increase Benztropine & Procyclidine blood levels by up to 40%.
- **Drug interactions with MAOIs:** Serotonin syndrome.

Warnings for paroxetine

➢ **Pregnancy**: **Risk category D**. The use of paroxetine during pregnancy should be avoided. Assessment of the risks versus benefits needs to be discussed with the patient.

➢ **MAOI**: Paroxetine may cause serotonin syndrome when it is used in combination with MAOIs. Paroxetine users require at least 2 weeks of a washout period before starting with MAOI and 7 days before switching from MAOI to paroxetine.

➢ **Elderly**: Paroxetine needs a dose reduction in the elderly.

- ➢ **Liver impairment**: Paroxetine needs a dose reduction in patient's with liver impairment.
- ➢ **Kidney impairment**: Paroxetine needs a dose reduction in patients with kidney impairment.
- ➢ **Activation of hypomania or mania** occurred in **1%** of paroxetine-treated patients compared to 0.3% of placebo-treated patients. In bipolar patients, the rates of manic exacerbation was 2.2% for the paroxetine-treated patients.
- ➢ **The incidence of seizures** is **0.1%** among the paroxetine-treated patients.
- ➢ **Discontinuation response** may develop when paroxetine is stopped abruptly. The most common discontinuation symptoms include dysphoric mood, agitation, anxiety, dizziness, irritability, paresthesias in the form of electric shock sensations, headaches, insomnia, emotional lability, lethargy and confusion. A gradual dose reduction is strongly recommended.
- ➢ **Hyponatremia** may develop subsequent to the use of paroxetine, especially in volume-depleted patients and in patients on diuretics. The symptoms of hyponatremia include headaches, reduced concentration, confusion, weakness and unsteadiness, which may lead to falls. Severe cases of hyponatremia may

result in seizures, hallucinations, respiratory arrest, coma and death.

➢ **Akathisia** was observed in paroxetine-treated patients and is characterized by an inner sense of restlessness, psychomotor agitation, and an inability to sit still. It is associated with significant distress.

➢ **Angle–closure glaucoma**: Paroxetine may have an effect on the pupil size resulting in mydriasis. Patients with narrow-angle glaucoma may experience increased intraocular pressure when treated with paroxetine.

➢ **Abnormal bleeding** was observed in patients using paroxetine. Concomitant use of warfarin, NSAIDs and aspirin may add to this risk.

Paroxetine overdose

Paroxetine is **rarely lethal in mono therapy overdose**. However, the concomitant use of paroxetine with alcohol and/ or with other central nervous depressants such as painkillers or benzo-diazepines may result in death caused by respiratory depression.

Overdose symptoms

The most common symptoms of paroxetine over dose are:

- somnolence
- nausea
- vomiting
- over sedation
- agitation
- confusion
- dizziness
- dilated pupils (mydriasis
- abnormal heart rhythm
- tachycardia
- bradycardia
- torsades de pointes
- hypertension
- stupor
- coma
- convulsions
- status epilepticus
- dystonia
- rhabdomyolysis
- myoclonus
- urinary retention
- acute renal failure
- hepatic dysfunction

How to manage paroxetine's overdosed patients

In general, there is no antidote for paroxetine overdose and the management is mainly supportive, aimed to maintaining respiration, pulse and blood pressure. In the event of a recent overdose with paroxetine, a stomach washout, possibly with activated charcoal, may help to eliminate the un-absorbed drug and is done with large–bore oro-gastric tube, maintaining appropriate airway protection. In most cases paroxetine overdose, requires to hospitalize the patient for at least 24 hours for intense observation.

Paroxetine references

1 Hiemke C, Haarter S, et al. Pharmacokinetics of SSRI. Pharmacol Ther 2000;85:11 – 28.

2 Jun-Sheng W, Hao-Jie Z. Bryan BG et al. Sertraline and its metabolite desmethylsertraline, but not Buproprion or its three major metabolites, have high affinity for P-gp. Biol Pharm Bull Feb 2008; 31(2): 231 – 234.

3 Baldwin DS, Hawley CJ, Abed RT et al. A multicentre double blind comparison of nefazodone and paroxetine in the treatment of outpatients with moderate to severe depression. J Clin Psychiatry 1996;57 (2):46-52.

4 Goldstein DJ, Lu Y, Detka M et al. Duloxetine in the treatment of depression: a double blind placebo controlled comparison with paroxetine. J Cl Psychopharmacology August 2004;Vol 24 (4) 389 – 399.

5 Montgomery SA, Dunbar G,. Paroxetine is better than placebo in relapse prevention and the prophylaxis of recurrent depression. Int Clin Psychopharmacology 1993;8: 189 – 195.

6 Claghorn JL, Feighner JP, et al A double blind comparison of paroxetine with imipramine in the long term treatment of depression. J Clin Psychopharmacology , 1993;13(2): 23-27.

Fourteen

Sertraline

Brand name: Zoloft

Mode of action

- **Sertraline is a Serotonin Reuptake Transporter (SERT) antagonist.**
- **Sertraline is a Dopamine Reuptake Transporter (DAT) antagonist.**
- **Dopamine D2 receptor:** The inhibition of the D2 receptors by sertraline may have some antipsychotic effects.
- **Sigma-1 receptor:** The inhibitory effects of sertraline on the Sigma1 receptors may be involved with its anxiolytic effects.
- **Anticholinergic (Ach)   Low affinity**
- **Histaminergic (H1):   Low affinity**
- **Adrenergic (α1):   Moderate affinity**

Pharmacokinetics of sertraline

Pharmacokinetics: Sertraline has **linear pharmacokinetics.** Thus, any dose change leads to a proportional change in the drug plasma levels. The higher the daily dose of sertraline, the higher the plasma level will get.

Peak plasma level (Tmax): 6-84 hours.

Absorption: Sertraline is absorbed slowly by the gastrointestinal system, and its absorption is accelerated by the presence of food.

Steady state: 7 Days.

Protein binding: 98%: mostly to albumin and to α1-glycoprotein.

Half-life (t ½): 26 – 32 hours for sertraline
        70 Hours for *desmethylsertraline* (sertraline's principal metabolite).

Bioavailability: Unknown

Metabolism: CYP 450 enzymes
- **2C9 (25%)**
- **3A4 (15%)**
- **2C19(15%)**
- **2D6 (5%)**

Sertraline is primarily metabolized by the liver via the enzymes of the CYP450 system. The principal pathway of metabolism is N-demethylation.

N-desmethylsertraline, which is the active metabolite, has a plasma terminal half-life of 62 to 104 hours, but it appears to be less active than its parent drug.

N-desmethylsertraline has a 50 times weaker effect on SERT than that of the parent drug; practically, this metabolites has no clinical effects.

Elimination: Urine 0.2%
Faeces 50%

How supplied

- Tablet: 25mg, 50mg, 100 mg
- Oral solution 20mg/ml

Dose range

- 50 mg – 200 mg for depression
- Doses of 200 mg a day may be required for OCD and bulimia

Clinical indications

- Major depressive disorder
- Panic disorder
- Obsessive compulsive disorder
- Premenstrual dysphoric syndrome
- Bulimia

How to treat with sertraline

- **For Depression & OCD**: Start with 50mg a day in a single morning dose. Wait at least two weeks to assess clinical improvement before increasing the dose in increments of 50 mg a week up to a maximum of 200mg a day.

- **For Panic disorder (PD), Social anxiety & Post-Traumatic Stress disorder (PTSD):** Start with sertraline 25mg a day, in order to avoid possible excitation and anxiety. Increase the dose in increments of 50mg after one week of treatment up to a maximum of 200mg a day. As a general rule, the higher the patient's anxiety is, the lower the starting dose of sertraline should be, and the slower the dose increase should be.

- **For premenstrual dysphoric disorder (PMDD)**: Start with sertraline 50 mg a day, a week before the upcoming menses cycle. However, in severe cases, patients need to take the medication throughout the menstrual cycle.

When and how to take medication

Preferably, sertraline should be used during the morning in order to avoid insomnia, which may be develop whenever sertraline is taken at night.

How to stop treatment: Due to its relatively long half-life, sertraline have lower incidence of withdrawal symptoms.

Sertraline discontinuation reaction

The most common symptoms of sudden discontinuation of sertraline are:
- nausea
- insomnia
- dizziness
- light-headedness
- vertigo
- nightmares and vivid dreams
- sensation of electric shock in the body
- anxiety

Side effects

Nervous system
- Activation (infrequent)
- Insomnia
- Agitation
- Restlessness
- Jitteriness
- Anxiety
- Tremor

- Worsening motor symptoms of Parkinson's disease
- Increased sweating/ flushing
- Headache
- Dizziness
- Seizures (rare)
- Cognitive slowing
- Reduced attention
- Apathy
- Emotional blunting
- Rash

Gastro intestinal
The GI side effects are common with sertraline and can develop within 30 minutes of drug ingestion. It is possible that the GI side effects are more likely the result of the direct effect of sertraline on the intestinal mucosa than to its peak plasma levels.
- Decreased appetite
- Upper gastrointestinal symptoms
- Nausea
- Vomiting
- Dry mouth
- Diarrhea or constipation
- Possible weight loss

Sexual
Sertraline like all other SSRIs, may affect sexual desire, performance and satisfaction.

- Decreased sex drive
- Delayed ejaculation
- Impotence
- Inability to reach an orgasm

Suicide

The FDA requires all antidepressants to carry a black box warning stating that antidepressant may increase the risk for suicide in persons under the age of 25 years. This warning is based on data suggesting that suicidal ideations and behavior has a 2 fold increase in children and in adolescents, and a 1.5 – fold increase in the 18 – 24 age group.

Sertraline side effects that requires immediate attention:

- Confusion
- Excitation
- Onset of seizure
- Yellow skin / eyes
- Severe allergic reaction
- Irregular heart beats
- Low blood pressure
- Bruising and bleeding (relatively rare)
- Induction of manic episode
- Activation of suicidal ideation and behaviour

Use during pregnancy: FDA risk category C. The use of sertraline in the last trimester of pregnancy may be associated with a higher incidence of respiratory distress and pulmonary hypertension, cyanosis, apnea, seizures, temperature instability, vomiting, hypoglycemia, hypotonia, hyperreflexia, tremor, irritability, constant crying and jitteriness, which may require prolonged hospitalization, tube feeding and respiratory support.

Use during lactation: Sertraline is secreted in the breast milk. Due to its unknown effects on the new born's normal growth and development, breast feeding should be avoided.

Avoid using sertraline in the following cases

- Proven allergy to sertraline
- Co-administration with MAOIs

Sertraline drug interactions

- **Drug interaction with Warfarin:** Increase bleeding.
- **Drug interaction with Tramadol, LSD:** Seizure.
- **Drug interaction with Lithium:** Nausea tremor.
- **Drug interaction with Pindolol & Propranolol:** Increase beta blockers blood levels.

- **Drug interactions with Pimozide, Thioridazine**: Increase antipsychotics blood levels.
- **Drug interaction with Alprazolam, Triazolam:** Increase BNZ blood levels.
- **Drug interaction with Buspiron:** Increase buspiron blood levels.
- **Drug interactions with Phenytoin**: Increase Phenytoin blood levels.
- **Drug interactions with MAOIs:** Serotonin syndrome.

Warnings for sertraline

➢ **Pregnancy**: Sertraline has an FDA risk category C. Try to avoid the use during pregnancy or breastfeeding. Assessment of the risks versus benefits must be discussed with the patient.

➢ **Myocardial infarction**: Sertraline is one of the few antidepressants that has been shown to be safe in the treatment of depression in patients with a history of myocardial infarction and angina.

➢ **Depressed pilots**: Sertraline was approved by the FAA for the treatment of depression in pilots.

- ➢ **Schizophrenic patients**: Sertraline has been shown to be effective in the treatment of depression in schizophrenic patients.
- ➢ **Children & adolescents**: Sertraline is effective in the treatment of depression in children and adolescents. Sertraline may increase the risk of suicidal thinking and behavior in children, adolescents and young adults aged 18-24. The use of antidepressants in this population must balance the risk of suicide with the clinical need. Careful monitoring of the patient's clinical worsening, and suicidality should also involve the family and all other caregivers.
- ➢ **Patients with increased prolactin levels**: Due to its minimal effect on prolactin, sertraline is effective in the treatment of depression in patients with high prolactin levels.
- ➢ **Hypomania & mania**: Activation of hypomania or mania occurred in 0.4% of sertraline treated patients.
- ➢ **Seizures**: No seizures were observed among 3000 patients treated with sertraline during sertraline FDA registration studies for MDD.
- ➢ **Discontinuation syndrome**: Discontinuation response may develop when sertraline is stopped abruptly. The most common discontinuation symptoms include dysphoric mood, agitation, anxiety, dizziness,

irritability, paresthesias in the form of electric shock sensations, headaches, insomnia, emotional lability, lethargy and confusion. A gradual dose reduction is strongly recommended.

> **Hyponatremia**: Hyponatremia may develop subsequent to the use of sertraline, especially in volume depleted patients and in patients on diuretics. The symptoms of hyponatremia include headaches, reduced concentration, confusion, weakness and unsteadiness, which may lead to falls. Severe cases of hyponatremia may result in seizures, hallucinations respiratory arrest, coma and death.

> **Angle–closure glaucoma**: Sertraline may have an effect on pupil size, resulting in mydriasis. Patients with narrow-angle-glaucoma may experience increased intraocular pressure when treated with sertraline.

> **Abnormal bleeding**: Abnormal bleeding was observed in patients using sertraline. Concomitant use of warfarin, NSAIDs and aspirin may add to this risk.

> **Uricosuric effect:** A mean decrease of 7% in serum uric acid was observed in patients on sertraline.

- ➤ **Asymptomatic liver enzyme increase**: Asymptomatic increases in liver enzyme was reported in 0.8% of patients using sertraline within the first 9 weeks of treatment. Liver enzymes increase in patients on sertraline is clinically insignificant.
- ➤ **Elderly**: Sertraline needs a lower dose in the elderly.
- ➤ **Liver impairment**: Sertraline need a lower dose in patients with liver impairment.
- ➤ **MAOI:** Sertraline requires a 2-week washout period before starting with a MAOI. After stopping a MAOI, wait 21 days before starting sertraline.

Sertraline overdose

Sertraline *is rarely lethal in mono therapy overdose*. However, the concomitant use of sertraline with alcohol and /or with other central nervous depressants such as painkillers, barbiturates and benzo-diazepines, may result in death caused by respiratory depression.

Overdose symptoms

The most common symptoms of sertraline over dose are:
- vomiting
- over-sedation
- somnolence

- dilated pupils
- abnormal heart rhythm
- tachycardia
- nausea
- tremor
- agitation
- coma
- seizures
- delirium
- hypertension / hypotension
- QTc prolongation
- syncope

How to manage sertraline's overdosed patients

In general, there is no antidote for sertraline overdose and the management is mainly supportive, aimed to maintaining respiration, pulse and blood pressure. In the event of a recent overdose with sertraline, a stomach washout, possibly with activated charcoal, may help to eliminate the un-absorbed drug and is done with large–bore oro-gastric tube, maintaining appropriate airway protection. In most cases sertraline overdose, requires to hospitalize the patient for at least 24 hours for intense observation.

Sertraline references

1 Hiemke C, Haarter S, et al. Pharmacokinetics of SSRI. Pharmacol Ther 2000;85:11 – 28.

2. Doogan DP, Caillard V et al. Sertraline in the prevention of depression. Br. J. Psychiatry 1992;160: 217-222.

3 Thase ME, Haight BR, Richard N. et al. Remission rates following antidepressant therapy with buproprion or SSRIs: A metaanalysis of original data from 7 randomized controlled trials. J. of Cl. Psy.2005; 66 (8): 974-981.

4 Hoehn – Saric R, Ninan P, Black D. et al. Multicenter double blind comparison of sertraline and desipramine for concurrent OCD and MDD. Arch. Gen. Psychiatry 2000;57 (1): 76-82.

5 Pohl R, Wolkow R, Clar C et al. Sertraline in the treatment of panic disorder: a double blind multicentre trial. Am J Psychiatry 1998;155: 1189-1195.

6 Jun-Sheng W, Hao-Jie Z. Bryan BG et al. Sertraline and its metabolite desmethylsertraline, but not Buproprion or its three major metabolites, have high affinity for P-gp. Biol Pharm Bull Feb 2008; 31(2): 231 – 234.

Fifteen

Trazodone

Brand name:
Molipaxin
Desyrel
Oleptro

Mode of action

- Trazodone is a weak antagonist of the Serotonin Reuptake Transporter (SERT).
- Trazodone is a strong *agonist* of the post-synaptic 5-HT 1A receptors.
- Trazodone a post-synaptic 5-HT2A receptor antagonist

- **Trazodone is a post-synaptic 5-HT2C receptor antagonist**.
- **Sigma-1 receptor:** The inhibitory effects of trazodone on the Sigma1 receptors may be involved with its anxiolytic effects.
- **Anticholinergic (Ach)   High affinity**
- **Histaminergic (H1):   Moderate affinity**
- **Adrenergic (α1):   Moderate affinity**

Pharmacokinetics of trazodone

Pharmacokinetics: Trazodone has **linear pharmacokinetics** and it does not appears to induce its own metabolism. Thus, any dose change leads to a proportional change in the drug plasma levels.

Peak plasma level (Tmax):
1 hour for trazodone
43 hours for the metabolite m-CPP

Absorption: Trazodone is well absorbed by the gastrointestinal system. However, the absorption of trazodone is *slowed by the presence of food* in the stomach, which may result in a delayed increase in trazodone plasma levels.

Steady state: 3-7 Days.

Protein binding: 95%: mostly to albumin and to α1-glycoprotein.

Half-life (t ½):   9 hours for trazodone.
4 -14 hoursfor m-CPP

Bioavailability: Unknown

Metabolism: CYP 450 enzymes **3A4**

Trazodone has an active metabolite called **m-CPP** which can accumulate to higher levels in the brain than in the blood. More than 75% of trazodone metabolites are excreted within 3 days.

Elimination: **Urine 80%**
Faeces 20%

How supplied

- Trazodone immediate release tablets 50mg, 100mg. 150mg
- Trazodone XR 150mg, 300mg

Dose range

- Trazodone 150 mg–400mg a day for depression
- Trazodone XR 150mg–375mg a day for depression

Clinical indications
- Major depression
- insomnia
- anxiety

How to treat with trazodon

- **For Major Depressive Disorder:** Start with trazodone 150mg in divided doses to be increased every 3 days to a maximum of 400mg in divided doses.

- For the treatment of depression with the extended release formula (trazodone XR), start with trazodone XR 150mg once a day to be increased every 3 days by 75 mg to a maximum dose of 375mg.

- **For insomnia:** Start with trazodone 50 mg in the evening, to be increased up to 100mg at bedtime.

When and how to take medication

Preferably take trazodone twice a day for the immediate release formulation and once a day at bedtime for the XR formulation. In general use the principle "start low and go slow", as patients can experience over-sedation the following day at the beginning of the treatment.

How to stop treatment

Although the incidence of withdrawal symptoms following trazodone cessation is relatively low, a slow tapering of trazodone is recommended.

Trazodone discontinuation reaction

The most common symptoms of sudden discontinuation of trazodone are:

- Irritability
- Agitation
- Dizziness
- Anxiety
- Confusion
- Headache
- Lethargy
- Insomnia
- Seizures
- Dysphoric mood
- Fever
- Fatigue
- Sweating
- Myalgia (muscle pain)
- Priapism

Side effects

Nervous system
- Drowsiness
- Lethargy
- Fatigue
- Weakness
- Dizziness

- Sedation
- Nausea
- Blurred vision
- Headache and worsening of migraine
- In coordination
- Tremor
- Disturbed concentration
- Disorientation
- Confusion
- Restlessness and agitation (rare)
- *Seizures* (more common in predisposed individuals, if occur, is often after sudden drug dose increase or after drug withdrawal).
- Stuttering
- Disturbance in gait
- Worsening of parkinsonism
- Rash (rare 1%)
- Hypotension
- Syncope
- bradycardia

Gastro intestinal

The gastro intestinal side effects of trazodone can develop within 30 minutes of drug ingestion and they are more likely the result of the trazodone's effects on serotonin uptake and its anticholinergic effects.

- *Decreased appetite*
- Weight gain

- Nausea
- Vomiting
- Dry mouth
- Glossitis
- Strange taste in mouth
- Constipation
- Gastritis

Sexual
- Increased libido
- Priapism
- Spontaneous orgasm with yawning
- Retrograde ejaculation
- Painful ejaculation
- Testicular swelling

Suicide

The FDA requires all antidepressants to carry a black box warning stating that antidepressant may increase the risk for suicide in persons under the age of 25 years. This warning is based on data suggesting that suicidal ideations and behavior has a 2-fold increase in children and in adolescents, and a 1.5–fold increase in the 18 – 24 age group.

Trazodone's side effects that requires immediate attention
- Priapism
- Confusion
- Excitation

- Onset of seizure
- Yellow skin / eyes
- Severe allergic reaction
- Irregular heart beats
- Hypotension
- Induction of manic or hypomanic episode
- Activation of suicidal ideation and behaviour especially in children and adolescents

Use during pregnancy: FDA risk category C. The use of trazodone in the last trimester of pregnancy may be associated with a higher incidence of respiratory distress and pulmonary hypertension, cyanosis, apnea, seizures, temperature instability, vomiting, hypoglycemia, hypotonia, hyperreflexia, tremor, irritability, constant crying and jitteriness, which may require prolonged hospitalization, tube feeding and respiratory support.

Use during lactation: Trazodone is secreted in the breast milk. Due to its unknown effects on the new born's normal growth and development, breast feeding should be avoided.

Avoid using trazodone in the following cases

- **Priapism**: In the event of male patients getting a painful erection which lasts longer than 4-6 hours, immediate urgent medical help is required. Priapism is often self-limited and reverses spontaneously. However, in 30%

of cases, it requires surgical intervention which may cause permanently impaired erectile function or impotence.

- **Persistent genital arousal in female:** Persistent genital arousal may be associated with trazodone use in female patients and it is similar to male priapism.
- **Cardiac arrhythmia**: Patients with pre-existing cardiac disease and cardiac arrhythmias should be closely monitored.
- History of seizure
- Proven allergy to trazodone.

Trazodone drug interactions

- **Drug interaction with Warfarin:** Increase bleeding.
- **Drug interaction with Tramadol, LSD:** Seizure.
- **Drug interaction with Digoxin:** Increase digoxin blood level.
- **Drug interaction with Carbamazepine:** Decrease trazodone blood levels.
- **Drug interactions with Zolpidem**: Sedation.
- **Drug interaction with Alprazolam:** Increase BNZ blood levels by 200%.
- **Drug interaction with Clozapine:** Increase clozapine blood levels.

- **Drug interactions with Phenytoin**: Increase Phenytoin blood levels.
- **Drug interactions with MAOIs:** Serotonin syndrome.
- **Drug interactions with Sildenafil:** Hypotension.

Warnings for trazodone

➢ **Pregnancy**: **Risk category C**. Try to avoid use during pregnancy or breastfeeding. Assessment of the risks versus benefits must be discussed with the patient.

➢ **Trazodone may cause an increase in suicidal risk in young adults**. The use of antidepressants in this population must balance the risks of suicide with the clinical need. Careful monitoring of the patient's clinical worsening is necessary, and monitoring for suicidality should also involve the family and all other caregivers.

➢ **Activation of hypomania or mania** may occur in trazodone treated bipolar patients. As trazodone may trigger mania in predisposed patients, it should be used cautiously in patients with a history of bipolar mood disorder.

➢ **Serotonin syndrome** may develop with trazodone use. Serotonin syndrome symptoms may include agitation, dizziness, hallucinations, delirium, seizures and coma along with autonomic instability which includes tachycardia, fluctuating blood pressure, flushing, hyperthermia, tremor, muscular rigidity, myoclonus, hyperreflexia, and incoordination. The concomitant use of trazodone with a MAOI may precipitate serotonin syndrome, which may be fatal.

➢ **MAOI:** After stopping trazodone a **7 day** washout period is needed before starting with a MAOI. After the MAOI was stopped, a **3 week** washout period is necessary before starting trazodone.

➢ **Priapism**: Painful erections lasting longer than 6 hours were reported in men taking trazodone. Priapism, if not treated promptly, may result in irreversible damage to the erectile tissue. Patients with anatomical deformation of the penis (such as cavernosal fibrosis, angulation or Peyronie's disease), as well as patients with sickle cell anemia, multiple myeloma or leukemia, should use trazodone with care as those conditions may predispose them to priapism. Patients who develop priapism lasting longer than 6 hour should seek emergency medical attention.

➢ **Hyponatremia:** Hyponatremia may develop subsequent to the use of trazodone, especially in volume depleted patients and in patients on diuretics. The symptoms of hyponatremia include headaches, reduced concentration, confusion, weakness and unsteadiness, which may lead to falls. Severe cases of hyponatremia may result in seizures, hallucinations respiratory arrest, coma and death.

➢ **Abnormal bleeding** was observed in patients using trazodone. Concomitant use of warfarin, NSAIDs aspirin may add to this risk.

➢ **Syncope:** Trazodone use was associated with syncope and hypotension. The concomitant use of trazodone with anti-hypertensive drugs may exacerbate hypotension.

➢ **Angle–closure glaucoma**: Trazodone may have an effect on pupil size resulting in mydriasis. Patients with narrow-angle glaucoma may experience increased intraocular pressure when treated with trazodone.

➢ **Cognitive & motor impairment**: Trazodone may cause somnolence and sedation, which may impair the mental and the physical ability required for the performance of hazardous tasks.

➢ **Discontinuation symptoms**: Trazodone discontinuation was associated with withdrawal symptoms of anxiety, agitation, and sleep disturbances. A gradual dose reduction is strongly recommended in order to avoid discontinuation symptoms.

➢ **Heart disease**: Trazodone is not recommended for use during the initial phase after having a myocardial infarction. Trazodone was associated with QT prolongation and isolated PVCs, tachycardia, syncope and torsade de pointes.

➢ **Liver impairment**: Trazodone should be taken in a lower dose in people with liver cirrhosis. Trazodone *must be avoided* in patients with liver insufficiency.

➢ **Alcohol abuse**: Trazodone is not recommended in patients abusing alcohol.

➢ **Kidney impairment**: Trazodone requires a dose adjustment (lower dose) in mild to moderate renal impairment.

➢ **Elderly:** Trazodone needs a dose adjustment (lower dose) in the elderly.

Trazodone overdose

Trazodone is relatively safe in mono therapy overdose with a rare incidence of fatalities. However, the concomitant use of trazodone with alcohol and with other central nervous depressants such as painkillers or benzo-diazepines may result in death caused by respiratory depression. The possible fatalities are often the result of cardio-respiratory arrest or the metabolic acidosis and hypoxia associated with status epilepticus.

Overdose symptoms

The most common symptoms of trazodone over dose are:

- Over-sedation
- respiratory arrest
- seizure
- abnormal heart rhythm – mainly tachycardia
- hypotension
- priapism
- vomiting
- delirium
- loss of consciousness

How to manage trazodone's overdosed patients

In general, there is no antidote for trazodone overdose and the management is mainly supportive, aimed to maintaining respiration, pulse and blood pressure. In the event of a recent overdose with trazodone, a stomach washout, possibly with activated charcoal, may help to eliminate the un-absorbed drug and is done with large–bore oro-gastric tube, maintaining appropriate airway protection. In most cases trazodone overdose, requires to hospitalize the patient for at least 24 hours for intense observation.

Trazodone references

1 Goldberg HL,Rickels K, Finnely R. Treatment of depression with a new antidepressant. J Clin Psychopharmacology. 1981; sup. 6 , 1:3s- 38s.

2 Nambudiri DE, Mirchandani IC, Young RC. Two more cases of trazodone related syncope in the eldely. J Geriatric Psychiatry Neurol 1989;2:225.

3 Dordling CM, Mischoulon D, Petersen TJ. Et al. The pharmacologic management of SSRI induced side effects: a survey of psychiatrist. Ann Clin Psychiatry 2002;14:143-147.

Sixsteen

Venlafaxine

Brand name:
Effexor
Ilovex
Venlor

Mode of action

- **Venlafaxine is a Serotonin Re-uptake Transporter (SERT) Antagonist.**
- **Venlafaxine is a Norepinephrine Re-uptake Transporter (NET) antagonist.**
- **Venlafaxine is a Dopamine Reuptake Transporter (DAT) antagonist.**

The inhibition of the SERT, NET and DAT transporters is dose-dependent. At lower doses, venlafaxine will block only SERT. At increasing doses, NET will be inhibited; DAT will only be inhibited at venlafaxine doses of 375mg and above. This effect is illustrated in Figure 16.1.

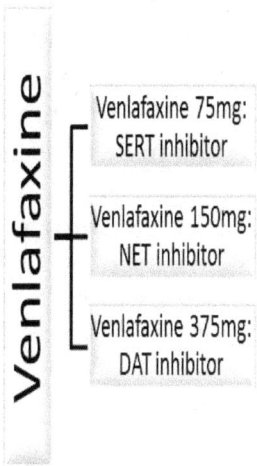

Figure 16.1 Dose-related effects of venlafaxine.

- **Anticholinergic (Ach)**   **Low affinity**
- **Histaminergic (H1):**   **Low affinity**
- **Adrenergic (α1):**   **Low affinity**

Pharmacokinetics of venlafaxine

Pharmacokinetics: Venlafaxine has **linear pharmacokinetics** and it does not appears to induce its own metabolism. Thus, any dose change leads to a proportional change in the drug plasma levels.

Peak plasma level (Tmax):
1-3 hours (immediate release),
6 hours (extended release)
2-6 hours (active metabolite ODV).

Absorption: Venlafaxine has **linear pharmacokinetics,** and it does not inhibit its own metabolism. Each dose increase of venlafaxine may lead to a proportionately greater increase in the venlafaxine plasma levels; thus, the higher the daily dose of venlafaxine, the higher the plasma level will get. Venlafaxine is well absorbed by the gastrointestinal system. More than 90% of the oral dose of venlafaxine will be absorbed into the blood circulation. Venlafaxine absorption is not affected by the presence of food or by the stomach pH.

Steady state: 3-7 Days.

Protein binding: **<35%**: mostly to albumin and to α1-glycoprotein.

Half-life (t ½): **3-7 hours** (Immediate Release)
15 hours (extended release)
9-13 hours (active metabolite ODV).

Bioavailability: 45%

Metabolism: CYP 450 enzymes **2D6**

Venlafaxine is metabolized by the isoenzyme **2D6** into an active metabolite: *O- Desmethylvenlafaxine* **(ODV),** which also has antidepressant effects which are as potent as those of the parent drug. The other metabolite of venlafaxine, *N-desmethylvenlafaxine,* has no clinical effects.

Elimination: **Urine 87%**
Faeces 15%

Patients with impaired kidneys should use 25% less venlafaxine, while patients who are on haemodialysis should use 50% less venlafaxine.

How supplied

- **Venlafaxine IR and XR capsules**: 37.5 mg, 75mg, 150 mg.

The Extended Release formula requires once a day dosing and has a lower incidence of side effects (particularly, lower incidence of nausea and other gastrointestinal discomfort).

Dose range

- For depression: 75 mg – 225 mg
- For generalized anxiety disorder: 150mg - 225mg once a day.

Clinical indications

- Major depression
- Generalised anxiety disorder
- Panic disorder
- Social anxiety disorder
- Post traumatic stress disorder
- Premenstrual dysphoric disorder (PMDD)

How to treat with venlafaxine

- **For depression:** start venlafaxine with a maximal daily dose of 75 mg, to be increased every 4 days, up to a maximum of 225mg a day. Continue with the higher dose until reaching the desired antidepressant efficacy. In severe cases, the maximum venlafaxine daily dose of 375mg needs to be used. This is attributed to the blocking of NET and DAT which only occur at higher doses of venlafaxine.

- **For generalized anxiety disorder:** start with 75mg a day to be increased weekly up to a maximum of 225mg a day.

When and how to take medication

Venlafaxine XR should be taken preferably in the morning as a once daily dose (Venlafaxine IR should be taken as a twice a day dose). The patient must avoid crushing or chewing the capsule as it will interfere with the drug absorption.

How to stop treatment

Due to its relatively short half-life, there is a need for a slow tapering of venlafaxine in order to avoid withdrawal symptoms. *It appears that venlafaxine's withdrawal symptoms are more common and more severe compared to other antidepressants.*

Venlafaxine discontinuation reaction

The most common symptoms of sudden discontinuation of venlafaxine are:

- Irritability
- Agitation
- Dizziness
- Nausea
- Electric shock sensations
- Diarrhea
- Muscle cramps
- Anxiety
- Confusion
- Nightmares
- Headache
- Lethargy
- Insomnia
- Seizures
- Dysphoric mood
- Seizures
- Dysphoric mood
- Fever
- Fatigue
- Sweating
- Myalgia (muscle pain)
- Priapism

Side effects

The nervous system: Venlafaxine is less activating compared to the SSRIs. The sedating effects of venlafaxine appear to be equivalent to SSRIs, but to a lesser degree than TCAs.

- Insomnia
- Nervousness
- Anxiety
- Restless leg syndrome
- Muscle spasm
- Tremor
- Hot flushes
- Headache
- Dizziness
- Blurred vision
- Seizures (rare, mainly associated with treatment discontinuation)
- Increased sweating
- Fatigue
- Somnolence
- Sedation
- Rash
- Hypertension

Cardiac

Increased blood pressure affects 2%-6% of the patients treated with venlafaxine, and it appears to be dose-related. Thus up to 12% of patients treated with venlafaxine at a mean dose of 350mg/day may develop hypertension.

Gastro intestinal : Venlafaxine often results in GI side effects, which can develop within 30 minutes of drug ingestion.

It appears that the gastro intestinal side effects of venlafaxine are more likely the result of the direct effect of venlafaxine on the intestinal mucosa than its effects on the CNS or plasma concentration.

Weight gain is a troublesome side effect associated with venlafaxine. Weight gain will develop slowly and can affect up to 16% of treated patients, and is comparable to weight gain with SSRIs.

- Decreased appetite
- Nausea
- Weight gain although weight loss is possible.
- Vomiting
- Dry mouth
- Diarrhea
- Constipation
- Gastritis

Sexual

The sexual-related side effects of venlafaxine will develop soon after the commencement of treatment and are relatively high but are comparable to those of SSRIs. Up to 30% of patients treated with venlafaxine can develop sexual impairments. The sexual side effects of venlafaxine are probably related to its effects on serotonin, and are more prominent in males than in females. Furthermore, it appears that the risk of sexual dysfunction is correlated with age and with higher venlafaxine doses.

- Decreased sex drive
- Delayed ejaculation
- Impotence
- Abnormal orgasm

Suicide

The FDA requires all antidepressants to carry a black box warning stating that antidepressant may increase the risk for suicide in persons under the age of 25 years. This warning is based on data suggesting that suicidal ideations and behavior has a 2 fold increase in children and in adolescents, and a 1.5 – fold increase in the 18 – 24 age group.

Venlafaxine side effects that requires immediate attention:

- Confusion
- Excitation
- Onset of seizure
- Yellow skin / eyes
- Severe allergic reaction
- Irregular heart beat
- Hypertension
- Induction of manic or hypomanic episode
- Activation of suicidal ideation and behaviour

Use during pregnancy: FDA risk category C. The use of venlafaxine in the last trimester of pregnancy may be associated with a higher incidence of respiratory distress and pulmonary hypertension, cyanosis, apnea, seizures, temperature instability, vomiting, hypoglycemia, hypotonia, hyperreflexia, tremor, irritability, constant crying and jitteriness, which may require prolonged hospitalization, tube feeding and respiratory support.

Use during lactation: Venlafaxine is secreted in the breast milk. Due to its unknown effects on the new born's normal growth and development, breast feeding should be avoided.

Special considerations when using venlafaxine

➢ **Narrow-angle glaucoma**: Venlafaxine can increase eye pressure due to its ability to potentiate the effects of norepinephrine (NE). Venlafaxine should be avoided in patients having un -controlled narrow-angle glaucoma.

➢ **Hypertension**: The Venlafaxine potentiating effects on norepinephrine (NE) can lead to increased heart rates and blood pressure. It appears that 2 – 6% of patients who are getting venlafaxine will experience an increased diastolic blood pressure; this appears to be dose-dependent.

- ➢ **PPHN**: Venlafaxine use was associated with persistent pulmonary hypertension of the new born (PPHN).
- ➢ **ECG**: Venlafaxine has no clinical effects on the ECG profile and on the QTc interval. It has been shown to be safe for the treatment of depression in patients with myocardial infarction and angina. However, in animal models, venlafaxine appears to be able to block the myocardial sodium channels; this has an unclear clinical implication.
- ➢ **Overdose fatalities**: There are several reports of fatal cardiotoxicity following venlafaxine overdose. Furthermore, overdose with venlafaxine may result in higher mortality rates than overdose with SSRIs (11).
- ➢ **Rhabdomyolysis**: There are several reports of rhabdomyolysis with the use of venlafaxine (12).
- ➢ **REM sleep**: Venlafaxine can supress REM sleep.
- ➢ **Bruxism**: Venlafaxine may cause bruxism.
- ➢ **Abnormal bleeding**: Venlafaxine may lead to abnormal bleeding and bruising. Concomitant use of warfarin, NSAIDs and aspirin may add to this risk.
- ➢ **Urinary hesitancy**: Venlafaxine's ability to potentiate norepinephrine (NE) can increase

urethral resistance, which might lead to urinary hesitancy.

➤ **Prostatic hypertrophy**: Venlafaxine should be used with caution in patients with prostatic hypertrophy due to possible urinary hesitancy and urinary retention.

Venlafaxine drug interactions

- **Drug interaction with Warfarin:** Increase bleeding.
- **Drug interaction with Tramadol, LSD:** Seizure.
- **Drug interaction with Fluvoxamine:** Increase venlafaxine blood level.
- **Drug interaction with Bupropion:** 3-fold increase in venlafaxine blood levels.
- **Drug interactions with Cimetidine**: 60% increase in venlafaxine blood levels.
- **Drug interaction with Zolpidem:** Delirium.
- **Drug interaction with Beta Blockers:** Increase venlafaxine blood levels.
- **Drug interactions with MAOIs:** Serotonin syndrome.

Warnings for venlafaxine

➤ **Pregnancy: Risk category C**. Try to avoid use during pregnancy or breastfeeding.

Assessment of the risks versus benefits must be discussed with the patient.

> **Suicide in children & young adults**: Venlafaxine may cause an increase in suicidal risk in young adults, and it carries a black box warning. Venlafaxine may cause a **5-fold increase** in suicidal ideations and suicidal behaviour in patients under 25 years of age. On the other hand, FDA analysis of suicide risk among adults using venlafaxine showed no significant difference from fluoxetine or placebo. Venlafaxine is contra indicated in children, adolescents and young adults due to the possible risk of suicide.

> **Serotonin syndrome**: Venlafaxine may cause serotonin syndrome. Serotonin syndrome symptoms include agitation, dizziness, hallucinations, delirium, seizures and coma along with autonomic instability, which includes tachycardia, fluctuating blood pressure, flushing, hyperthermia, tremor, muscular rigidity, myoclonus, hyperreflexia, and incoordination. The concomitant use of venlafaxine with a MAOI may precipitate serotonin syndrome which may be fatal.

> **MAOI**: Venlafaxine requires a *1 week washout period* before starting treatment with a MAOI. After a MAOI is stopped a 3-

week washout period is required before starting venlafaxine.

➤ **Renal impairment**: Venlafaxine requires a lower dose in mild to moderate renal impairment.

➤ **Liver insufficiency**: Venlafaxine should be avoided in patients with liver insufficiency.

➤ **Alcohol abuse**: Venlafaxine is not recommended in patients abusing alcohol, due to the effects on the liver.

➤ **Mania & hypomania**: Venlafaxine may trigger mania in predisposed patients. It should be used cautiously in patients with a history of bipolar mood disorder.

➤ **Elderly**: Venlafaxine needs a lower dose when it is used in the elderly.

Venlafaxine overdose

Overdose with venlafaxine can be lethal. Data from the U.K suggests that venlafaxine overdose carries a higher rate of lethality when compared with SSRI overdose. Furthermore, the concomitant use of venlafaxine with alcohol and with other central nervous depressants such as painkillers or benzo-diazepines may result in death caused by respiratory depression. The possible fatalities are often the result of cardio-respiratory arrest or the metabolic acidosis and hypoxia associated with status epilepticus.

Overdose symptoms

The most common symptoms of venlafaxine over dose are:

- vomiting
- over-sedation
- agitation
- seizures
- abnormal heart rhythm-tachycardia
- hypertension

How to manage venlafaxine's overdosed patients

In general, there is no antidote for venlafaxine overdose and the management is mainly supportive, aimed to maintaining respiration, pulse and blood pressure. In the event of a recent overdose with venlafaxine, a stomach washout, possibly with activated charcoal, may help to eliminate the un-absorbed drug and is done with large–bore orogastric tube, maintaining appropriate airway protection. In most cases venlafaxine overdose, requires to hospitalize the patient for at least 24 hours for intense observation.

Venlafaxine references.

1.Nemeroff, CB, Willard, L. Et al: venlafaxine and SSRI: Pooled remission analysis. New research poster presented at the 156th APA annual meeting , San Francisco, CA, May2003; 17-22.

2 Schmitt A.B, Bauer, M. et al. Differential effects of venlafaxine in the treatment of MDD according to baseline severity. European Archives of Psychiatry and Clinical Neuroscience, 2009;259, 329 – 339.

3 Kornstein, S.G, Mao, .Y et al. Escitalopram versus SNRI antidepressants in the acute treatment of major depressive disorder. CNS Spectrums, 2009;14(6), 326-333.

4 Davidson J.R, Meoni P. et al,. Archieving remission with venlafaxine and fluoxetine in major depression: its relationship to anxiety symptoms. Depression and anxiety, 2002;16(1), 4-13.

5 Thase, M.E, Entsuah, et al. Relative antidepressant efficacy of venlafaxine and SSRIs: sex- age interaction. Journal of woman Health, 2005;14, 6009-616.

6 Papakostas G.I, Thase M.E, Fava M. et al. Are antidepressant drugs that combine serotonergic and noradrenergic mechanisms of action more effective than the selective serotonin reuptake inhibitors in treating MDD? A meta analysis of studies of newer agents. Biological Psychiatry 2007;62, 1217 – 1227.

7 Benkert,O., Grunder, G, Wetzel, H et al. A randomized double blind comparison of a rapid escalating dose of venlafaxine and imipramine in inpatients with MDD and melancholia. Journal of Psychiatric Research, 1996;30(6), 441 – 451.

8 Rickels K., Pollack M., Sheehan D. et al. Efficacy of XR venlafaxine in non – depressed outpatients with GAD. Am. J. Psychiatry 2000;157: 968 – 974.

9 Allgulander C, Hackett D, Salinas E et al. Venlafaxine ER in the treatment of GAD: twenty – four week placebo – controlled dose – ranging study. Br J. Psychiatry 2001;179:15-22.

10 Allgulander C., Mangano R, Zhang J, et al Efficacy of venlafaxine ER in patients with SAD. A double blind, placebo – controlled , parallel group comparison with Paroxetine. Human Psychopharmacology 2004;19: 387 – 396.

11 Flanagan, R.J,. Fatal toxicity of drugs used in psychiatry. Human Psychopharmacology, 2008;23 (Supp. 1), 43 – 51.

12 Wilson A. D, Howell, C, & Waring, W. Venlafaxine ingestion is associated with rhabdomyolysis in adults: A case serie. J. of Toxicological Sciences, 2007;32 (1), 97 – 101.

13 Clerc GE, Ruimy P, Verdeau- Pailes J. A double blind comparison of venlafaxine and fluoxetine in patients hospitalized for MDD and melancholia. Int. Clin. Psychopharmacol. 1994; 9:139-143.

14 Septien- Velez L, Pitroski B., Padmanahan SK et al, . A randomized double blind, placebo controlled trial of desvenlafaxine succinate in the treatment of MDD. Int. Clin. Psychopharmacol. 2007;22:338-347.

15 Lieberman, D.Z, Montgomery, SA, Tourian, K et al. A pooled analysis of two placebo – controlled trials of desvenlafaxine in major depressive disorder. Int. Clin. Psychopharmacol.2008; 23 (4), 188 – 197.

Seventeen
Vilazodone

Brand name:
Viibryd

Mode of action

- Vilazodone is a Serotonin Reuptake Transporter (SERT) antagonist
- Vilazodone is a partial agonist of 5-HT1A receptors

Pharmacokinetics of vilazodone

Pharmacokinetics: Vilazodone has **linear pharmacokinetics which are dose- dependent.** Thus, any dose increase leads to a proportional increase in the drug plasma levels.

Peak plasma level (T_{max}): 4-5 hour

Absorption: Vilazodone is well absorbed by the gastrointestinal system. The administration of vilazodone with food will *increase* it oral bioavailability by 160% and its AUC by 85%. However, if vomiting occurs within 7 hours of ingestion, vilazodone's absorption is decreased by 25%.

Steady state: 3 Days.

Protein binding: **96%-99%** mostly to albumin and to α1-glycoprotein.

Half-life (t ½): 25 hours

Bioavailability: 72%

Metabolism: CYP 450 enzymes **3A4**

Elimination: **Urine 80%**
The presence of mild to moderate renal impairment as well as mild to moderate liver impairment does not affect the vilazodone clearance.

How supplied

- Tablets 10mg, 20mg, and 40mg.

Dose range

10mg - 40mg a day for depression

Clinical indications

- Major depression

How to treat with vilazodone

- **For Depression:** Start with vilazodone 10mg a day, ingested preferably with food, for seven days, followed by an increase to 20mg for an additional seven days, and then increase to 40mg a day. The maximum dose should be lowered to a 20mg a day when it is co-administered with CYP 3A4 inhibitors, such as the antifungal ketoconazole, protease inhibitors, macrolides and verapamil.

When and how to take medication

Preferably take vilazodone at bedtime to avoid over-sedation. In general, use the principle "start low and go slow" as patients can experience over-sedation the following day at the beginning of the treatment.

How to stop treatment

It is highly recommended to taper vilazodone slowly in order to minimize the emergence of withdrawal symptoms, which usually develop within the first 2 weeks of treatment cessation. A 50% dose reduction every third day is recommended. In the event of the patient developing withdrawal symptoms, re-instate the previous dose, and once the symptoms disappear, start reducing the vilazodone dose in a smaller proportions and over a longer period of time.

Vilazodone discontinuation reaction

The most common symptoms of sudden discontinuation of vilazodone are:

- irritability
- agitation
- dizziness
- anxiety
- confusion
- headache
- lethargy
- insomnia
- seizures
- dysphoric mood
- fever
- fatigue
- sweating

- myalgia (muscle pain)
- electric shock sensation

Side effects

Nervous system

- dizziness
- somnolence
- paresthesias
- tremor
- insomnia
- abnormal dreams
- restlessness
- fatigue
- feeling jittery
- headache and worsening of migraine
- ***seizures***.

Gastro intestinal

The gastro intestinal side effects can develop within 30 minutes of drug ingestion, and they are more likely the result of the effects of vilazodone on the serotonin uptake.

- Nausea
- Diarrhea
- Dry mouth
- Vomiting
- Dyspepsia
- Flatulance
- Gastroenteritis
- Heartburn

- Increased appetite

Sexual

The incidence of sexual side effects with vilazodone are relatively low.

- decreased libido
- erectile dysfunction
- abnormal orgasm
- delayed ejaculation

Suicide

The FDA requires all antidepressants to carry a black box warning stating that antidepressant may increase the risk for suicide in persons under the age of 25 years. This warning is based on data suggesting that suicidal ideations and behavior has a 2 fold increase in children and in adolescents, and a 1.5 – fold increase in the 18 – 24 age group.

Vilazodone side effects that requires immediate attention

- Confusion
- Excitation
- Onset of seizure
- Yellow skin / eyes
- Severe allergic reaction
- Irregular heart beat
- Hypotension
- Induction of manic or hypomanic episode

- Activation of suicidal ideation and behaviour especially in children and adolescents

Use during pregnancy: FDA risk category C. The use of vilazodone in the last trimester of pregnancy may be associated with a higher incidence of respiratory distress and pulmonary hypertension, cyanosis, apnea, seizures, temperature instability, vomiting, hypoglycemia, hypotonia, hyperreflexia, tremor, irritability, constant crying and jitteriness, which may require prolonged hospitalization, tube feeding and respiratory support.

Use during lactation: Vilazodone is secreted in the breast milk. Due to its unknown effects on the new born's normal growth and development, breast feeding should be avoided.

Avoid using vilazodone in the following cases

- Patients with known allergy to vilazodone
- Patients with a history of seizure

Vilazodone drug interactions

- **Drug interaction with Warfarin:** Increase bleeding.
- **Drug interaction with Tramadol, LSD:** Seizure.
- **Drug interaction with Ketoconazole:** Increase vilazodone blood level.

- **Drug interaction with Carbamazepine:** Decrease vilazodone blood levels.
- **Drug interactions with Tamoxifen**: Decrease vilazodone blood levels.
- **Drug interaction with Triptans:** Serotonin syndrome.
- **Drug interaction with Verapamil:** Increase vilazodone blood levels.
- **Drug interactions with MAOIs:** Serotonin syndrome.
- **Drug interactions with Grapefruit juice:** Decrease vilazodone metabolism.

Warnings for vilazodone

➤ **Pregnancy**: **Risk category C**. Try to avoid use during pregnancy or breast feeding. Assessment of the risks versus benefits must be discussed with the patient.

➤ **Seizure risk**. Vilazodone was not associated with increased seizure activity. However, patients with a history of seizure require caution when using vilazodone, as well as patients with an increased predisposition to have seizures, such as brain damage, as well as alcohol abusers.

➤ **Vilazodone may cause an increase in suicidal risk in young adults**. The use of antidepressants in this population must balance the risk of suicide with the clinical need. Careful monitoring of the patients clinical worsening is necessary. Evaluation for suicidality should also involve the family and all other caregivers.

➤ **Activation of hypomania or mania** may occur in vilazodone-treated bipolar patients. As vilazodone may trigger mania in predisposed patients, it should be used cautiously in patients with a history of bipolar mood disorder

➤ **Serotonin syndrome** may develop with vilazodone use. Serotonin syndrome symptoms may include agitation, dizziness, hallucinations, delirium, seizures and coma along with autonomic instability, which includes tachycardia, fluctuating blood pressure, flushing, hyperthermia, tremor, muscular rigidity, myoclonus, hyperreflexia and incoordination. The concomitant use of vilazodone with MAOIs, triptans, TCAs, lithium, fentanyl, tramadol, tryptophan, buspirone and St. John's Wort may precipitate serotonin syndrome.

➤ **Renal impairment**: Vilazodone does not require a lower dose in mild to moderate renal impairment.

➢ **Liver impairment**: Vilazodone does not require lower dose in patients with liver impairment.

➢ **Alcohol:** Vilazodone is not recommended in patients abusing alcohol.

➢ **Withdrawal reaction**. Vilazodone use may result in a withdrawal reaction, prevention of which requires a slow reduction of vilazodone dose. The onset of withdrawal symptoms is attributed to vilazodone's relatively short half-life. The withdrawal symptoms of vilazodone can develop as early as the second day of the drug's sudden discontinuation and may persist for several days. The most common withdrawal symptoms are nausea, dizziness, insomnia, anxiety, tension and headache.

➢ **MAOI:** Vilazodone's combined use with a MAOI may be fatal. Vilazodone requires **7 day** washout period before starting with a MAOI. A **3 week** washout period is needed after the MAOI was stopped before starting with vilazodone.

➢ **Weight**: Vilazodone was not associated with weight gain.

➢ **Abnormal bleeding:** The use of vilazodone and SSRIs may be associated with increased risk of bleeding. The concomitant use of aspirin, NSAIDs and warfarin may add to this risk. Bleeding has ranged from ecchymosis, hematoma, epistaxis and petechiae to life-threatening hemorrhage.

➢ **Hyponatremias**: No cases of hyponatremia were reported with the use of vilazodone.

Vilazodone overdose

Vilazodone was not lethal in mono therapy overdose. The concomitant use of vilazodone with alcohol and with other central nervous depressants such as painkillers or benzo- diazepines may result in death caused by respiratory depression. The possible fatalities are often the result of cardio-respiratory arrest and the metabolic acidosis and hypoxia which are associated with status epilepticus.

Overdose symptoms

The most common symptoms of vilazodone over dose are:
- Lethargy
- Restlessness
- Hallucinations
- Disorientation
- Serotonin syndrome

How to manage vilazodone's overdosed patients

In general, there is no antidote for viazodone overdose and the management is mainly supportive, aimed to maintaining respiration, pulse and blood pressure. In the event of a recent overdose with vilazodone, a stomach washout, possibly with activated charcoal, may help to eliminate the un-absorbed drug and is done with large–bore oro-gastric tube, maintaining appropriate airway protection. In most cases vilazodone overdose, requires to hospitalize the patient for at least 24 hours for intense observation.

Vilazodone references

1 Rickels K, Athanaasiou M, Robinson DS et al. Evidence for efficacy and tolerability of vilazodone in the treatment of MDD; a randomized, double-blind,placebo-controlled trial. J Clin Psychiatry. 2009;70(3);326-333.

Suggested reading

Psychopharmacology

Julien RM, Advokat C, Comaty JE. A primer of drug action. Worth Publishers 2011.

Leonard Lichtblau. Psychopharmacology Demystified. Delmare Cengage Learning. 2011.

Meyer JS, Quenzer LF. Psychopharmacology. Drugs, the brain and behavior. Sinauer Associates, Inc.2005.

Harvey RA, Champe PC. Lippincott's Illustrated Reviews, Pharmacology Lippincott Williams & Wilkins 2006.

Nestler EJ, Hyman SE, Malenka RC. Molecular Neuropharmacology. A foundation for clinical neuroscience.McGraw Hill Medical 2009.

Rang HP, Dale MM,Ritter JM, Moore PK. Pharmacology. Churchill Livingstone 2003.

Kalyna Z. Bezchlibnyk-Butler, J. Joel Jeffries. Clinical handbook of Psychotropic drugs. 14 edition, Hogrefe & Huber 2004.

PG Janicak, SR Marder, MN Pavuluri. Principles and Practice of Psychopharmacotherapy. Fifth edition. Lippincott Williams & Wilkins, 2011.

Treatment

1 Brook S. Physician Guide to Antidepressants. CreateSpace, 2013.

2 Stahl SM. Stahl's Essential Psychopharmacology. Cambridge University Press 2008.

3 Stahl S.M. The prescriber Guide. Cambridge University Press. 2011.

4 Schatzberg AF, Nemeroff C B. Essentials of clinical psychopharmacology. American Psychiatric Publishing Inc. 2006.

5 Papakostas GI, Fava M. Pharmacotherapy for Depression and Treatment Resistant Depression. World Scientific 2010.

6 Stein DJ, Lerer B, Stahl SM. Essential Evidence based Psychopharmacology. Cambridge University Press. 2012.

7 Kennedy SH, Gorwood P. Successful Management of Major Depressive Disorder. Evolving Medicine, Ltd 2012.

8 Stern TA, Fricchione GL, Cassem NH, Jellinek MS, Rosenbaum JF. Handbook of General Hospital Psychiatry. Saunders Elsevier 2010.

9 Kennedy SH, Lam RW, Nutt DJ, THase ME. Treating Depression Effectively.Martin Dunitz, informa healthcare, 2007.

Internet

www.dailymed.nlm.gov/dailymed/lookup

wwww.preskorn.com

www.medicine.iupui.edu/flockart

www.drugs.com

Appendix 1

P- Glycoprotein (P-gp)

P-glycoproteins (P-gp), are glycoproteins encoded by the ABC1 gene. They are trans-membrane proteins with 6 trans- membrane domains and an additional large cytoplasmic domain containing ATP-binding sites.

The main function of P-gp is to transport a variety of substrates across the cellular membranes. They function to protect the body from harmful substances by active transportation of hydrophobic substances across the cell membrane.

The P-gp are efflux transporters located in various organ cells such as the liver, the kidneys, the adrenal glands, the placenta, the gonads, the biliary system, intestines and the brain.

P-gp activity requires energy provided by the ATP, and is capable of regulating the absorption and excretion of drugs and other substances from various body organs.

P-gp is subject to induction and inhibition similar to that of the P450 enzymes. The P-gp glycoprotein located in the gut can act as a gatekeeper and block the absorption of harmful substances and drug from the gastrointestinal system.

P-gp mechanism of action

The P-gp substrate binds to the P-gp simultaneously with one ATP molecule.

The hydrolysis of the ATP shifts the substrates into a position to be excreted from the cell.

The release of the phosphate from the ATP molecule occurs simultaneously with the release from the substrate. The remaining ADP then is also released from the P-gp and a new ATP molecule attaches and resets the cycle. There are more than 100 genetic variations of the P-gp glycoprotein due to a single nucleotide polymorphysm.

Woman appears to have lower hepatic P-gp levels than man, which may explain why some drugs are metabolized more efficiently by woman. The p-gp significantly affects drug pharmacokinetics by its ability to regulate the drug transport across the cell membrane. For example, increased intestinal expression of P-gp can reduce the absorption of drugs, which are P-gp substrates resulting in their lower plasma levels.

The P-gp can also facilitate the transport of compound out of the brain, across the blood brain barrier.

P-gp substrates

Methotrexate, mitomycin, vincristine, amiodarone, atorvastatin, dilitiazem, digoxin, lovastatin, nadolol, pravastatin, propranolol,timolol, quinidine, verapamil, clarithromycin, erythromycin, fluoroquinolones,
quinine, rifampin, indinavir, ritonavir, cyclosporine, cimetidine, lidocaine, loperamide, morphine,

P-gp inhibitors

Amiodarone, diltiazem, cyclosporine, itraconazole, verapamil, verapamil, clarithromycin, erythromycin, ritonavir, cyclosporine, nifedipine, propafenone, ketoconazole, mefloquine, ofloxacin

P-gp inducers

Dexamethasone, phenobarbital, rifampine, St. John's wort,

Antidepressants absorption and elimination from the body organs are also influenced by the P-gp system. Follows a list of antidepressants and their effect on the P-gp:

Antidepressants P-gp substrates

Agomelatine, amitriptilinr, citalopram, fluoxetine, fluvoxamine, mirtazapine, paroxetine, sertraline, venlafaxine.

Antidepressants P-gp inhibitors

Citalopram, duloxetine, fluoxetine, fluvoxamine, imipramine, paroxetine, sertraline, trazadone, venlafaxine.

Antidepressants P-gp inducers
Unknown

Appendix 2

Follows is a list of CYP 450 substrates, inhibitors and inducer

1A2 substrates

Duloxetine, clozapine, caffeine, acetaminophen, methadone, mirtazapine, olanzapine, propranol, tacrine,theophylline, bupropion, agomelatine, amitriptilline, chlorpromazine, clozapine, imipramine, melatonin, zolpidem.

1A2 inhibitors

Cimetidine, fluvoxamine, moclobemide, ticlopidine, midefradil, fluoroquinolone, perphenazine.

1A2 inducers

Omeprazole, tobacco, barbiturates, carbamazepine, modafinil, phenytoin.

3A4 substrates

Alprazolam, amiodaron, aripiprazole, buspirone, codeine, cyclosporine, diltiazem, estrogen, erythromycin, fentanyl, amitriptyline, bupropion, chlorpromazine, citalopram, clomipramine, clonazepam, clozapine, diazepam, donepezil,galantamine, haloperidol, midazolam, mirtazapine, modafinil, quotepine, reboxetine, risperidon, trazadon, zolpidem, zopiclone, venlafaxine.

3A4 inhibitors

Cimethidine, dexamethasone, diltiazem, ketoconazole,ritonavir, verapamil, saquinavir, fluconazole, fluoxetine, fluvoxamine, paroxetine, reboxetine, perphenazine.

3A4 inducers

Barbiturates, carbamazepine, phenytoine, St. John's Wort, rifampin, modafinil, topiramate.

2C19 substrates

Agomelatine,amitriptyline, carbamazepine, citalopram, clomipramine diazepam, escitalopram, fluoxetine, moclobemide, phenytoin, trimipramine, tranylcypromine.

2C19 inhibitors

Fluvoxamine, moclobemide,modafinil, topiramate, escitalopram,cimethidine, ketoconazole, omeprazole,phenytoin, tranylcypromine,fluoxetine, imipramine.

2C19 inducers

Rifampin, carbamazepine,St. John's Wort.

2C9 substrates

Agomelatine, amitriptillyne, bupropion, fluoxetine, lamotrigine, phenytoin, valproic acid, fluvastatin, celecoxid, losartan, rosiglitazone, warfarin, tolbutamide.

2C9 inhibitors

Fluoxetine, fluvoxamine, modafinil, valproic acid, amiodaron, d- propoxyphene, disulfiram, fluconazole, fluvastatine, miconazole, sulphaphenazole, zafirlukast.

2C9 inducers

St. John's Wort, carbamazepine,phenytoin, rifampin,secobarbital

2D6 substrates

Amphetamine, venlafaxine, aripiprazole, atomoxetine, beta blockers, thioridazine,risperidone, codeine, haloperidone, clozapine, desipramine, donepezil, duloxetine, mirtazapine, perphenazine, tamoxifen, tramadol, trazadone, morphine oxycodone,zuclophentixole,iloperidone,ondasterone atomoxetine, tropisetron, amphetamine, metoclopramide, promethazine, phenacetine, dexfenfluramine.

2D6 inhibitors

Fluoxetine, sertraline,paroxetine, citalopram, bupropion,cimetidine, haloperidol, methadone, moclobemide, quinidine, ritonavir, cinacalcet, duloxetine, terbinafine, thioridazine, risperidone, St. John's Wort, chlorpromazine, hydroxyzine, diphenhydramine, cocaine ranitidine.

2D6 inducers

Dexamethazone, rifampicin, glutethimide

2B6 substrates

Bupropion, ifosfamide, tamoxifen, ketamine, cyclophosphamide, nevirapine, artemisin, efavirenz sibutramine, propofol, arachidonic acidlauric acid, estrone, ethinylestradiol, testosterone.

2B6 inducers

Carbamazepine.

Antidepressants historical overview

Since the late 1950s, the treatment of major depressive disorder (MDD) with antidepressants gained momentum and replaced other treatment modalities such as Freudian psychoanalysis, which had previously dominated the psychiatric management of MDD.

The increase knowledge of neuroanatomy, neurophysiology and neuro-pharmacology along with the advances in drug development and manufacturing led to a boom in the development of new antidepressants.

Imipramine was the first Tricyclic Antidepressant (TCA) to be developed. Imipramine was presented at the first International Congress of Neuropharmacology held in Rome in September 1958. Imipramine showed encouraging results in the treatment of 46 patients with depressive psychosis.

During the same period, several reports in the medical literature emerged, suggesting that an anti-tuberculosis agent called iproniazid was shown to have mood elevating properties.

Soon after, a number of drugs inhibiting the monoamine oxidase enzymes (MAO inhibitors, or MAOI) were developed and investigated for possible antidepressant efficacy.

The TCAs and MAOI antidepressants showed good antidepressant efficacy.

The antidepressant effects were related to their ability to block the norepinephrine and serotonin re-uptake transporters (in the case of TCAs), and to irreversibly block the MAO enzyme (MAO inhibitors), which resulted in increased levels of serotonin and norepinephrine in the brain.

For 30 years, the MAOIs and TCAs dominated the antidepressant markets despite having serious tolerability and safety issues which will be thoroughly discussed in the relevant chapters.

Nevertheless, over the years, the TCAs and MAOIs were reasonably effective in treating depression. However, their severe side effects seriously affected patient's adherence to treatment. Many patients were unable to continue with the recommended treatment with TCA and MAOI and either terminated early the proposed treatment regimens or used sub-therapeutic doses.

The need to develop new antidepressants with improved tolerability and improved efficacy resulted in the development of the SSRIs which were introduced into the market in the mid-1980s.

The newly developed SSRIs gained enormous popularity due to their simplified use (once-a-day dose), better tolerability and improved safety with overdose, and yet with comparable efficacy to the older TCAs.

However, despite reasonable efficacy and improved tolerability, the severe sexual-related side effects that developed with the SSRIs, as well as the need for an at least 2-week waiting period before any treatment response, resulted in the necessity of development of alternative antidepressants.

During the 1990s, new antidepressants were introduced into the market with the promise of having better tolerability, safety in overdose and faster antidepressant action.

The Serotonin Norepinephrine Reuptake Inhibitors (SNRI) had dual action on the serotonin reuptake transporters as well as on the norepinephrine re uptake transporters. They provided some hope for faster and better antidepressant efficacy combined with improved tolerability.

However, that the SNRIs had better and faster efficacies was somewhat due to marketing success rather than actual clinical proof. Thus, the search for better and faster antidepressant continued.

Along came bupropion capable of inhibiting the dopamine reuptake transporters (DAT), and agomelatine, the first antidepressant to inhibit melatonin receptors (with effects on the 5-HT2C receptors and the circadian rhythms).

However, despite brilliant marketing, even these new antidepressants had severe side effects and similar efficacy to that of the older antidepressants. This is where antidepressant medications stand today. Given that the array of drugs is still unsatisfactory, the search for improved antidepressant medications continues.

It appears that future research is moving beyond the Serotonin Reuptake Transporters (SERT), the Norepinephrine Reuptake Transporters (NET) and the Dopamine Reuptake Transporters (DAT) and towards targeting the post-synaptic serotonin receptors located on the serotoninergic neurons in the amygdala and in the limbic system.

The current focus of research is on the post-synaptic 5-HT1A – agonists, 5 –HT 2A antagonists, 5-HT2C antagonists and 5 –HT 1D antagonists.
These newly targeted receptors appear to be involved with depressive mood, anxiety, insomnia and agitation and may produce a more potent and faster response, along with an improved tolerability and safety profile.

The hope is that the new medications will have quicker onset and safer action, which will ultimately improve adherence to treatment and will consequently improve remission rates and functionality of depressed patients.

Categories of antidepressants

TCAs

The TCAs are antidepressants, that were developed in 1957 after the discovery by the Swiss psychiatrists, Roland Kuhn, of the calming effects of imipramine on agitated depressed patients. All the TCAs have a basic three-ring structure, and all have a broad range of receptor affinity, which is responsible for their low tolerability and poor safety in overdose and can be lethal in overdose.

In addition, the TCAs have a strong affinity for the adrenergic $\alpha 1$, histaminergic H1, and acetylcoline Ach receptors, which results in their strong anticholinergic side effect profile. These anticholinergic symptoms include dry mouth, blurred vision, constipation, and urinary retention as well as excessive sedation, weight gain and hypotension.

SSRI (Selective Serotonin Reuptake Inhibitors)

The SSRIs were developed in the early 1980s. The class currently includes five members who share a similar inhibitory effect on the serotonin reuptake transporter (SERT). Follows is a list of the serotonin reuptake transporter inhibitors according to their affinity to SERT.

- Paroxetine   (Highest affinity)
- Citalopram
- Fluvoxamine
- Sertraline
- Fluoxetine   (Lowest affinity)

Due to the lack of a direct correlation between the SSRIs plasma levels with their antidepressant effects, the SSRI antidepressant response rate is unaffected by daily dose increases. This results in a flat dose response curve. The lack of a dose response may be related to the SSRI's ability to block at least 80% of the serotonin re-uptake transporters at the lowest dose which has an antidepressant effect.

In addition to the inhibitory effect on SERT, all SSRIs are capable of blocking the 5-HT1A auto receptor which is situated on the pre synaptic nerve cell. These receptors have an on/off function for the production and the release of serotonin from the pre synaptic nerve cell.

Blocking the pre synaptic 5-HT1A receptors will enhance the production and the release of serotonin from the pre synaptic nerve cell, while the activation of the pre synaptic 5-HT1A receptors will significantly reduce the amount of serotonin released by the pre synaptic nerve cell.

Most SSRIs have a milder side effect profile compared to the older TCAs generation. Furthermore, it appears that most SSRIs produce an array of side effects which seems to be slightly more tolerable than those seen with the TCAs.

The most common side effects of the SSRIs class include anxiety and agitation, headache, nausea, gastrointestinal discomfort, increased bowel motility, GI cramps and diarrhea. The SSRIs also have strong sexual side effects, which include reduced sex drive, anorgasmia and delayed ejaculation.

The SSRIs sexual-related side effects are very common and affect at least a one-third of treated patients and will often reduce a patient's adherence to treatment. Fortunately, most of the SSRIs side effects are temporary and often tend to reduce over time.

Serotonin & Norepinephrine Reuptake Inhibitors (SNRIs)

The SNRI class is a relatively new addition to the antidepressant family. The SNRIs have a strong affinity for both the serotonin and the norepinephrine reuptake transporters.

The first SNRI agent to gain FDA approval for the treatment of major depression was venlafaxine. Several years later, three additional agents gained access to the antidepressant market.

The SNRI timeline is as follows:
- 1993 Venlafaxine
- 2004 Duloxetine
- 2008 Desvenlafaxine
- 2009 Milnacipram (Not approved by the FDA)

The SNRIs gained popularity amongst prescribers due to their proven antidepressant efficacy, good tolerability and relative safety in overdose.

Most SNRIs have an ability to inhibit the serotonin reuptake transporters (SERT) as well as the norepinephrine reuptake transporters (NET). This dual effect on SERT and NET may be responsible for the better antidepressant efficacy.

It appears that the current clinical data suggests that the SNRIs have a higher remission rate compared to the SSRIs. Moreover, venlafaxine seems to have better efficacy at higher doses, which is probably due to its ability to block both the serotonin and the norepinephrine reuptake transporters as well as the dopamine re uptake transporters (DAT).

It is speculated that the ability of the SNRIs to increase brain dopamine levels is more prominent in the prefrontal cortex, which is one of the key areas involved with mood.